FACE THE FACTS

A Book About the Facts of Life for
Young People

By James A. Aderman

Northwestern Publishing House
Milwaukee, Wisconsin

Scripture taken from the
HOLY BIBLE, NEW INTERNATIONAL VERSION
Copyright © 1973, 1978, 1984 International Bible Society
Used by permission of Zondervan Bible Publishers.

Library of Congress Card 92-80013
Northwestern Publishing House
1250 N. 113th St., Milwaukee, WI 53226-3284
© 1992 by Northwestern Publishing House
Printed in the United States of America
ISBN 0-8100-0425-9

DEDICATION

To Rachel, Rebekah, and Sarah
I Love You

CONTENTS

1. The Adventure Begins 1

2. You Are Sexual 7

3. Here's What It's About.......................................14

4. Not Everyone Sees It That Way..........................24

5. Once upon a Time 39

6. The Male Half of the Reproductive System.......53

7. The Female Half of the Reproductive System ...62

8. Monthly Preparations for New Life....................70

9. It Can Make You Sick...79

10. Here It Comes..85

11. Solo Sex 93

12. Pregnancy and Contraception.........................103

13. More Than Growing: Maturing.........................113

14. Same-Sex Sex...126

15. Sex That Perverts..141

16. Sex That Hurts..149

17. God, Thank You I'm Sexual..............................158

PREFACE

On the day I turned thirteen, I found a book on my pillow. It was entitled, *From Teens to Marriage*. My mother wrote on the cover page,

> *This is my special gift to you. I pray you will read it slowly, devour and absorb every word, and digest it not only from the human side, but with a Christian outlook as well.*
>
> *There are many, many things in this book you won't really understand until you are an adult and a married man. But your next few years will be full of obstacles, happiness, fears, and decisions. Perhaps in some way this book will help you.*
>
> *Never forget to ask for guidance from above. Let that be your first thought. And always remember that your mom and dad will always help and stand by you if you will only come to us with your problems and worries.*
>
> *Good luck in your teen years to come.*

*And have a grand, glorious time becoming
an adult. Let God be your constant companion and friend. He will never fail you.*

I turned to that book many times over the next
years. Somehow it seemed less threatening to
research my questions about growing into adulthood
on my own. I knew I could trust my parents' answers
to my questions about sex, but I often found it hard to
bring up the subject. It was easier to talk with my
friends about sex, but I wasn't sure I could trust their
answers. I found answers in *From Teens to Marriage*
for most of my questions and comfort for most of my
concerns. For me it wasn't the perfect book, but it
was adequate.

I don't anticipate that this book will be the perfect
book either. Even the people I asked to review these
pages did not agree on what needs to be said to teens
about sexuality and what should be withheld until
later. But I do anticipate that Christian teens will be
assisted in their walk with Jesus through this book.
That's been my prayer as I penned these pages and as
they are published. I trust my God will honor my
request.

Trying to understand the changes I was going
through as a teen often confused and frustrated—if
not frightened—me. It's worse today for teens. Television, rock stars, movies, sports heroes, teen magazines often portray a grossly twisted view of human
sexuality. Each year one out of ten teenage girls
becomes pregnant. Homosexuality is flaunted as an
alternate lifestyle. Other sexual perversions are openly
broadcast. Sexually transmitted diseases are at epi-

demic levels among teens. Only a minority are still virgins by the time they reach 18. Respected educators, politicians, and even religious leaders assume that the normal child will be sexually active, so they structure programs to help teens practice "safe sex."

I felt sick writing about some of the issues this book addresses. *From Teens to Marriage* never came close to dealing with many of those topics. But we can't shelter our teens from the sexual cesspool that swirls around us. And we can't deny it's there. What we can do is arm our teens with the truth of God's word and will, build them up in their appreciation for God's grace, and motivate them to live for their loving Lord.

Consequently, the purpose of this book is fourfold.

1. That the teens who read this book will grow in their gratitude to God for his goodness and grace, in their appreciation of his wisdom in designing humans as he has, and in their desire to live lives that thank him.

2. That the teens who read this book will recognize that the changes they are going through mark the normal path everyone travels to reach adulthood. Everyone's path is different, but that, too, is normal.

3. That the teens who read this book are equipped to meet the special challenges to sexual purity which grow out of a culture that has made a god of sex.

4. That the teens who read this book will have a resource of accurate and biblical information that will serve them well from early puberty through early adulthood.

Thirty years ago my mother had no way of knowing that her inscription in my special birthday gift would ever find its way into another book for teens. But I find that her prayer for me back then is exactly my prayer for those who read this book now.

This is my special gift to you. I pray you will read it slowly, devour and absorb every word, and digest it not only from the human side, but with a Christian outlook as well.

Acknowledgements

A number of special friends have helped review this book. I am greatly appreciative of their time, suggestions, encouragement, and prayer. They include:

Miriam Festerling
Robert Fischer
Sandy Greenfield
John Juern
Janet Lindemann
Pamela Merten
Kenneth Proeber
Kimberly Volkmann
Peggy White
JoAnn Wilken
Stuart Zak

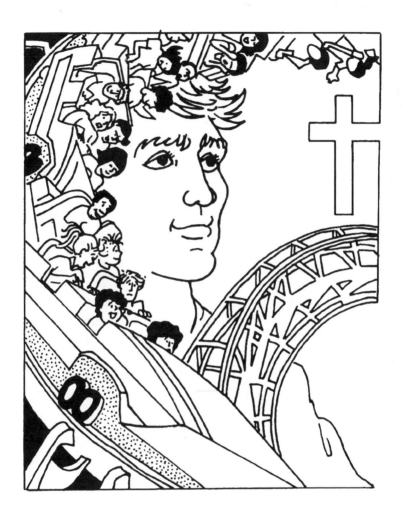

1.

THE ADVENTURE BEGINS

Suddenly my feet danced in the air. I was grabbed around the neck and lifted high above the ground. Steel-like fingers were strangling me. A long gory claw, glistening in the moonlight, choked and shook me. The monster looked at me through demon-red eyes. I screamed but nothing came out. "This is a dream!" I shouted to myself. "I want to wake up!"

Sound familiar? We all have nightmares from time to time. Scary books or movies usually help set the mood. When I was growing up, movies about ghosts always guaranteed me a restless night's sleep.

But then, so did some parts of my adolescence. Unfortunately, those sections of my teen years had to be lived through; I couldn't escape by waking myself up.

Adolescent Ups and Downs

Don't misunderstand. My teen years contained a lot more pleasant times than nightmares. I fondly remember the close friendships I had with "the guys." I was thrilled to notice the girls in my class were getting shapes where they didn't have shapes before. I enjoyed being treated as more grown up by my parents.

But there were embarrassing times, like the time my face was splattered with acne right before the biggest date of my life, like the time my voice crackled uncontrollably during forensics, and like the time I ripped the seam out of the back of my shorts during phy ed. I didn't quite understand everything that was happening to me during my teens. Where those sexual thoughts about girls were coming from and what to do about them confused me. Sometimes I couldn't figure out who I was. Sometimes I felt miserable about myself. A lack of coordination that stopped me from being much of an athlete didn't do anything for my self-esteem. And I often struggled with guilt feelings about things I wasn't responsible for—and for things that I was.

Adolescence (the time when we change from child to adult) is like that for everyone: a roller-coaster mixture of happiness and confusion, security and loneliness, a desire to march forward into the unknown and a white-knuckled clinging to what you know. Some of that happens because we don't have enough information. Some of it happens because we have misinformation. And some of it can't be escaped even if we have enough accurate information. Those ups and downs are built into making the transition to adult.

That's why it's important for you to know what's taking place within you and your friends as you become adults. Otherwise adolescence can become a frightening nightmare from which you wish you could awaken.

Talking about Adolescence

I hope that you and your parents have long talks about your growing into an adult. Sometimes parents can seem out of touch with reality, but they'll be an important source of information through your teen years if you'll let them.

Sometimes, though, parents are uneasy about sharing their thoughts on being a teenager. Some of that may have to do with their own insecurities and problems during adolescence. Some of it may be because they feel they lack information. Some of it comes with the recognition that society is different today from what it was twenty years ago (or more), when your parents were teens. Some of it may be motivated by being unsure how you will take their advice. (Chapter Thirteen, "More than Growing: Maturing," will have more on communicating with your parents.)

Any help your parents might offer you may also be affected by your own queasiness about discussing with them the changes you are experiencing. If you think you might not be normal or if you think you might have done or thought something terribly wrong, you probably won't be too ready to tell Mom and Dad, right?

When I was in junior high, I was afraid to tell my parents that there were lustful thoughts troubling me. I felt guilty as "all get out" about those thoughts, but also pleasured by them. And that made me feel even guiltier. That's why I was afraid to tell them. I just knew my parents would think I was weird, maybe insane, if they ever found out. So I kept quiet.

I hope that's where this book will be helpful to you. I pray that it will enable you to face the facts of how God has designed us to grow up, to face the facts of what it means to mature, to face the facts of life.

I intend to write this book as a friend might write to you. I'd like it to be the kind of knowledgeable friend I felt I needed during my early teen years. I've done a bunch of studying to make sure that what I tell you is accurate. I also have some stories to tell you about my teen years and the experiences of others that I think you will be able to relate to.

Be patient with me, though. Some of the things I'm going to share with you may be hard to understand. Some things you may have to think about for a long time before they'll make sense to you. And not everything in the book will be information you need right now. That's OK. Use what interests you. If there is a chapter or a part of a chapter that tells you something you don't think you need to know right now, it's perfectly all right to skip it. At some later point, you'll probably find those parts of the book will answer the questions you have then. I'd like you to think of this volume as a handbook you'll read now but also pull off your shelf from time to time over the next years.

No matter how often you read this book, though, there is something important I want you to come away with—a fact you really need to face. I want to assure you that what is happening to you as you grow into adulthood is what's supposed to be happening. Many changes will take place in your emotions, your thinking, and certainly also your body. I want you to know they are coming—or if they're already happening, that it's OK. In fact, it's more than OK.

The changes we all go through on our journey into adulthood are part of God's beautiful plan for our growth and development as human beings. The changes along the way may make us uncomfortable from time to time, but the end result shows us how much our God loves us and how wise and wonderful he is.

That's another fact I want to impress on you

throughout this book: you have a God who loves you more than you'll ever be able to appreciate. He proved that when he sent his Son to become one of us. But there's more. When he allowed his Son to be punished on the cross for all the sins we'll ever commit, he certified his love for us. And there's still more. That Son rose from the dead three days later, just as he said he would. That's your guarantee that your sins are forgiven, heaven is your destiny, and the wise and powerful God who created and rules the universe is your loving Father. The God who has done all of that for you won't let you down during adolescence.

My soul finds rest in God alone; my salvation comes from him. He alone is my rock and my salvation; he is my fortress, I will never be shaken. One thing God has spoken, two things have I heard: that you, O God, are strong, and that you, O Lord, are loving. (Psalm 62:1,2,11,12)

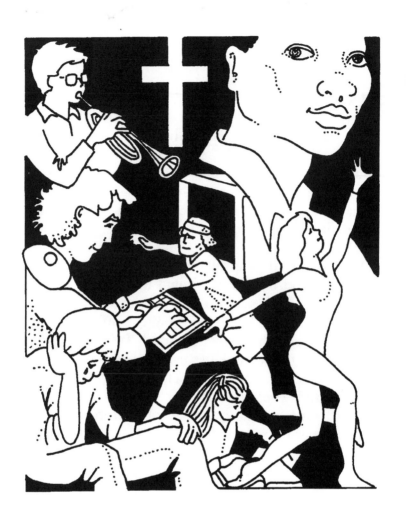

2.

YOU ARE SEXUAL

You are sexual.

It's true. You are sexual.

I wasn't very happy to face that thought somewhere around seventh grade. I had been satisfied living in a world inhabited by a bunch of boys with whom I could play baseball, football, and other sports, hike, and build tree forts. And, yes, there were girls in my world, too, (giggly things with long hair who seemed to cry a lot), but I didn't spend much time thinking about them. The beginning of adolescence changed all of that.

It was more than a mite confusing to discover that another world existed all around the world I and my male friends had built. It contained girls—and I mean girls! I realized that they were pretty, mysterious, and attractive, and they smelled good. I didn't want to throw away the world I was used to, but I didn't want to miss out on this new world either. Life was so much simpler B.C.—before curls.

Sure enough. Like my ancestors before me, I discovered that I was sexual.

Sexuality: a Definition

You are sexual, too. But did you notice? I said you are sexual. That's not the same as sexy or wanting to be sexually active. Better let me explain.

Being human means being sexual. We can't escape it. You are either a male or a female. You have a gender, a sex. That makes you a sexual being. That makes you what God planned you to be. Remember: "Male and female he created them" (Genesis 1:27).

Allow me to get a little philosophical for a few paragraphs. I know you can handle that.

Sexuality is different from sex (sex in the sense of intercourse). Sexuality is all the ingredients that go into our sexual nature. Sexual activity is only part of that sexual nature. Sexuality includes our gender and its characteristics: our body size and shape, our way of thinking and acting, our reproductive organs, our emotional make-up, the way males and females relate to each other, and, yes, how men and women make love with each other. Like a tangle of string in the back of a junk drawer, our sexuality and our humanness are completely knotted together.

We are sexual beings not only when we feel sexual urges, but in everything we do and experience. We can't turn it on or off. It is part of us. Our sexuality as a male or female will express itself in the way we choose clothes, play tennis, get angry, do homework, get along with our friends, and dream about the future. It is much more than the facts of life, much more than being able to reproduce. Our sexuality touches everything in our lives.

You are sexual. Pleasure has a lot to do with our sexuality. God has designed us so that when we use our sexuality properly we will experience pleasure. Sometimes we might get the impression that, since sexuality can be misused and can hurt us, the pleasure that goes with being sexual must be evil. That's not so.

When God created your body, he gave you a wide range of physical sensations. You can smell, see, feel, hear, and taste. Each of your senses, when used in the right way, gives pleasure. Good food pleases us.

Beautiful scenery pleases us. Upbeat, uplifting music pleases us. But too much good food will make us sick; admiring the beauty of the sun can blind us; painfully loud music can rob us of hearing. So our sexuality when properly used will bring us great pleasure, but when abused will cause us great pain.

Embarrassed about Our Sexuality

You are sexual. There's nothing wrong with admitting that. In fact, to be healthy, we must face that fact. And that means thinking about our sexuality: what it means, how we can expect it to shape our lives, how to make use of it. Thinking about our sexuality (and remember that's different than thinking sexually stimulating thoughts) is important. It's just as important as thinking about your digestive system and the kinds of food it needs to power your body.

But for some people thinking about—and learning about—their sexuality is extremely difficult. Some people feel ashamed of who they are, the gender God has made them, the things of which they are capable as a male or female. Their embarrassment about sexuality gets in the way of dealing with it. There are a number of reasons some people refuse to acknowledge their sexuality. Among them are:

1. Sometimes negative feelings are caused by the way their parents talked about their birth. Perhaps they were unwanted children, who were viewed as a burden and a hardship rather than as a blessing and joy.

2. Sometimes negative feelings develop because peo-

ple aren't given enough opportunities to be around others of their own gender or because those they are around are very poor models.

3. Sometimes negative feelings spring from the way their parents treated people of their gender, and every time their mother or father ridiculed their gender they felt worse about who they were.

4. Sometimes people feel ashamed of their sexuality because they were made to feel guilty and dirty for their natural curiosity about sex. Perhaps as youngsters they got undressed with children of the opposite sex and their parents punished them severely rather than understanding that behavior as curiosity.

5. Sometimes people have negative feelings about their sexuality because human sexuality was never respected in their homes. If they were sexually abused as a child, that would certainly have a negative effect on their view of sexuality.

6. Our sexuality is even shaped by the pet names our parents give to genitals (sex organs). If a person had parents whose names for genitals gave the impression that sexuality was repulsive, ugly, or terrible, that person might regard his sexuality negatively.

Created as Sexual Beings

Whether we are comfortable dealing with it or not, we are still sexual beings. We can't escape it, and we shouldn't want to. Our sexuality is a gift to us from our loving God.

You are sexual. That's the way God has designed all human beings. From the day he created Adam and Eve, there has been human sexuality. Sexuality is a gift of God's love and wisdom. Because God loves you and knows what's best for you, he made you male or female. It's because of God's grace and wisdom that he gave you, not just a masculine or feminine body, but masculine or feminine emotions, desires, and ways of looking at life.

More than that, Jesus came to earth, lived, died, and rose again to rescue from hell, not just your body, but also the soul that lives in your male or female body. He became your Savior not just to provide you with heaven, but to help you recognize your great worth in God's eyes. Because of that worth you'll now want to use your sexuality to praise him and benefit yourself. Oh, and there's more. Since you know how important you are to God, you'll also want to respect the sexuality of those with whom you share this planet.

Because we Christians are grateful for Jesus, we'll want to use our sexuality according to God's guidelines. That certainly includes listening to the things God tells us about sexual activity, marriage, and having children. Our power source for using our sexuality properly is God's Spirit as he works in our lives through his word and sacraments. That's the reason I'm going to be encouraging you throughout this book to plug into that power source. Bible study with others, personal Bible reading, Scripture memorization, frequent communion, and regular weekly worship are all ways to plug in. Make those ways a regular part of your life.

Father, I thank you for making me a sexual being. I have to admit that sometimes that makes me feel uneasy about myself. There are a lot of confusing things that go with being male or female. But I know that it is all according to your plan—and that plan is the best plan. I know that you love me more than I could ever understand, because you sent your Son to be my Savior and to make me your child. That's why I can thank you for making me a sexual being even though I don't always feel thankful. Please keep reminding me of how wise you are and how much you love me so I never forget to thank you for the way you direct me through life and on to life with you.

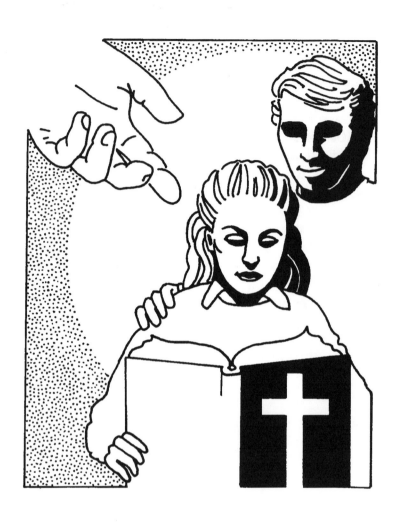

3.

HERE'S WHAT IT'S ABOUT

Put an X on the line below where you believe sexual intercourse is best described.

1————————————50——————————100
Dirty   Beautiful

We said in the last chapter that knowing what God's word says about our sexuality is essential to understanding who we are and to using our sexuality as he intends. That means there's no better way to find out how dirty or beautiful sexual intercourse is than to check out what God tells us in the Bible.

God's Word on Sex

Let's start right in the beginning—back when God created human beings. Remember how God said, "Let us make man in our image, in our likeness, and let them rule over the fish of the sea and the birds of the air, over the livestock, over all the earth, and over all the creatures that move along the ground"? Genesis 1:26-28 goes on, "So God created man in his own image, in the image of God he created him; male and female he created them. God blessed them and said to them, 'Be fruitful and increase in number; fill the earth and subdue it. Rule over the fish of the sea and the birds of the air and over every living creature that moves on the ground.'"

Notice a couple of things: God created a two-gender system; "male and female he created them." And he didn't just suggest, he commanded that they "Be fruitful and increase in number." Those words were more than a stern order barked out by a drill sergeant kind of God. Look at the words right before that command. God "blessed" them when he commanded, "Be fruitful and increase." Humankind's ability to reproduce is a gift from God intended to make men and women happy, blessed.

And do you remember God's evaluation of his creation? In the final verse of the Bible's first chapter we find God surveying everything he had made over the last six days. His survey included a man and a woman who, among other things, were sexual creatures. We're told, "God saw all that he had made, and it was *very good*" (Genesis 1:31).

Adam and Eve turned out just like the universe: *very good*. They turned out the way our perfect God intended. They were suited for each other. Each brought to their relationship some things that the other did not possess. They were designed to help each other, to care for each other, and to give pleasure to each other. Sexual intercourse was to be a normal, wonderful, beautiful part of their relationship.

That there was nothing sinful about their sexual relationship is clear when God tells us, "The man and his wife were both naked, and they felt no shame" (Genesis 2:25). It was only after sin came into the world that sexuality, now messed up by sin, came to be viewed as shameful. But as long as we use God's gift of sex according to his plan, there is no shame or dirtiness. There is only beauty and good.

Listen to what Psalm 139:14 says about our bodies: "I praise you because I am fearfully and wonderfully made; your works are wonderful, I know that full well." We are to praise God for providing our souls with such magnificent bodies in which to live. That praise includes properly using our ability to reproduce and to experience all sorts of pleasure,including sexual pleasure. (We'll have more to say about the pleasure of sexual activity in a couple of paragraphs.)

Our sexuality and sexual intercourse are a beautiful gift from the Lord. God created them and called them "very good." When we use those gifts properly, they are a blessing to us. "For everything God created is good, and nothing is to be rejected if it is received with thanksgiving, because it is consecrated by the word of God and prayer" (1 Timothy 4:4,5).

But how do we use the gift of sexual intercourse properly? Just what is God's purpose in giving human beings that gift?

Sexual Intercourse's Purpose

I got a ski parka for Christmas when I was thirteen. It was the best present I received that year. I was a ski jumper back then, and I knew that parka would make me look great as I flew through the air.

But one day I wore it while helping push a car out of a snowbank. By the time the car was free, I was dirty. Some of the spots never did come out. And I never looked as good again on the ski hill.

God has given us something much better than any ski parka, the beautiful gift of sex. But if we fail to take care of his gift, its beauty will be spoiled, like my parka. That's why we need to know why God has provided us with the ability to enjoy sexual activity. There are three reasons:

1. Companionship

In Genesis 2:18 God describes his reason for making human beings male and female: "The Lord God said, 'It is not good for the man to be alone. I will make a helper suitable for him.'" Adam was all alone. God determined that was "not good." He had a plan that would end loneliness for Adam. He would "make a helper suitable for him."

This "helper suitable" was not just someone of the opposite sex, but Adam's lifelong companion, his wife. Adam quickly caught on. When he first laid eyes on Eve, he exclaimed, "This is now bone of my bones and flesh of my flesh; she shall be called 'woman,' for she was taken out of man" (Genesis 2:23). From Adam's reaction to seeing Eve, it's also apparent why God created Eve from Adam's rib. He wanted to impress Adam and Eve with the closeness their relationship was to have. Adam and Eve were to solve each other's "not good" situation of loneliness.

Sexual intercourse between a husband and a wife is one of the ways that loneliness is eased. In Genesis 4:1 we're told, "Adam lay with his wife Eve, and she became pregnant." God used a wonderful word in this verse to describe the sexual relationship Adam and Eve enjoyed. The Hebrew word translated "lay with" actually means "know." Sexual relations enable a man and a woman to know each other, to know not just what each other's bodies look like, but to sense and experience one another's manhood or womanhood. This is knowing at its most intimate depth. It's that ability to "know" someone that takes away loneliness at this deepest of levels.

That's why it makes so much sense to limit sexual relations to marriage. Moses says in Genesis 2:24 that "a man will leave his father and mother and be united to his wife, and they will become one flesh." Becoming "one flesh" is not just a way of describing the closeness that happens when a husband and wife have sex. It describes the oneness which allows husbands and wives to accept each other for the people God has made them and to feel enough at ease with each other (because they trust each other) to show each other who they really are.

But unless a man and woman have made a marriage commitment to each other (that, come what may, they will never leave each other), that kind of deep-down acceptance cannot happen. Without a marriage commitment, both the man and the woman will hold back in their relationship with each other, afraid to reveal who they really are for fear the other will not accept them. Without the promises of lifelong faithfulness in marriage, sexual relations will not communicate commitment and love in the deepest sense. Rather they will only communicate how each person is selfishly using the other for his/her own sexual pleasure. Casual sex says, "I'm in this for what I can get out of it. If you don't please me, I'm leaving." That's not love. That only adds to one's loneliness; it can't take the loneliness away.

Someone I know who was sexually active as a teenager admitted to me,

It has to do with trust, really. I trusted him. I trusted him when he told me, "I love you." He trusted me when I said the same. We trusted our emotions when they said, "It's OK. Show each other how much you care." So I gave him my body and he gave me his.

It was the beginning of what we thought would be a romantic dream come true. Come to find out, it was the beginning of a nightmare of mistrust and, finally, abandonment. Instead of setting us free to express our love to each other, sex made us slaves of each other. I thought if I said "No" I'd lose him. He thought he couldn't say "No" because he had gotten a taste of what was now hard for him to live without. We were both trapped in what we didn't understand.

Instead of joining our hearts as one, sex slowly tore our hearts apart. I resented him for taking me for granted, for demanding all of me. He resented me for not freely giving in. Communication ceased. Understanding each other's feelings was not part of us anymore. My world as I once knew it collapsed around me. Nothing was as it had been. I came to realize I'd never be able to reclaim the loss.

When our relationship died, so did a part of me. The physical joining of our bodies powerfully worked at destroying my life. Even now as I relive the memory, I am surrounded by darkness and intense loneliness. I don't want to stay here for too long. The memory still is painful—and terrifying. All because I trusted a lie.

2. Pleasure

Sexual intercourse feels good. That's part of the blessing God has built into our sexuality. Married couples want to please each other through their sexual activity.

The goodness of the pleasure of sexual relations within marriage is clear from passages like Deuterono-

my 24:5. One of God's Old Testament rules is recorded there. It says, "If a man has recently married, he
must not be sent to war or have any other duty laid on
him. For one year he is to be free to stay at home and
bring happiness to the wife he has married." Young
Hebrew men were exempted from the military draft
for one year after their wedding date in order to
"bring happiness to" their new wives. That would certainly include having sex with them.

The Song of Solomon is something of a marriage
manual. It describes what God intends marital love to
be like. Some Christians are surprised to find such
"racy" material in the Bible, but sex within God's
guidelines is created to be stimulating, fun, and pleasurable. It's no wonder God has commanded, "The
husband should fulfill his marital duty to his wife, and
likewise the wife to her husband" (1 Corinthians 7:3).

However, some people think that because sex
makes us feel good, anyone should feel free to experience it. But thinking that way isn't right. Snorting
cocaine or shooting heroin might make us feel great,
too. But those drugs would also cause terrible damage.
The fact that something feels good doesn't mean we
should experience it—especially when God tells us to
stay away from it until we're in the right situation.

3. Creation of Children

There's another reason for sexual relations: children. Isn't it wonderful how God designed human
reproduction to result from a husband and a wife
showing committed love for each other? That also
tells us a lot about the love a mother and father show
their children.

Children are intended to be part of a marriage. The Lord made that clear when he gave his directives to the first husband and wife team. "God blessed them and said to them, 'Be fruitful and increase in number; fill the earth.'" Having children is a blessing from God. Christian husbands and wives dare not decide they can say to God, "You can keep your blessings, Lord, we've got other plans." (Read more about this in Chapter Twelve, "Pregnancy and Contraceptives.")

How unfortunate it is, however, that children come into the world when they are not the result of a man and woman's commitment to lifelong love for each other. How deprived that child will be while growing up. What a burden that man and woman must bear for allowing their desire for pleasure to hurt another human being, the child they produced.

Guidelines to Benefit Us

God has designed sexual relations to help take away our loneliness, to give us pleasure, and to produce children who are loved. So you see, our God is not being an old grinch when he restricts sexual relations to marriage. He is showing us how much he loves us. He's saying, "Here's a wonderful gift I've created for you. But to enjoy it fully, this is the way you must use it."

Many great blessings, when used in the wrong way, cause great harm. That reminds me of a story about a man who used to be called Righty. His wife gave him a chain saw for a birthday present. Righty hadn't ever used a chain saw and didn't have any instructions for using it. He used it once. Now Righty is called Lefty.

God gives us instructions for using our sexuality. He

has shared those rules with us, not to take our fun away, but to enable us to have the most pleasure with none of the pain. We can trust those directives for at least two reasons:

1. He made us. He should know how we best work.

2. He loves us. Jesus is the proof of that. How could a God who sacrificed his only Son so we could be forgiven, ever tell us to do anything or not to do something that's going to hurt us?

But treating our sexuality properly isn't easy—even with the Spirit's help. You'll discover why in the next chapter.

What a loving God you are, Father! Thanks. It's no wonder your angels in heaven constantly sing, "Hallelujah! Praise the Lord!" I see your love in the gift you have given me in being able to experience sexual intercourse. I also see your love in the instructions you have given me about when and how to use that gift. You want only good things to happen in my life. Your instructions about using your gift of sex will help that to be the case. What a wonderful God you are! But then, you are also the God who has punished your own Son so I could be your child. You are wonderful! I love you!

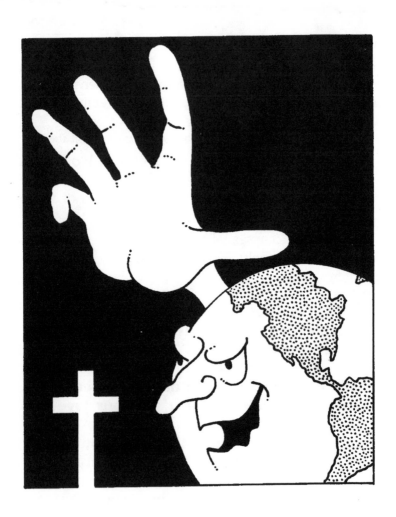

4.

NOT EVERYONE SEES IT THAT WAY

"Hey, did you hear? Marian Franks is pregnant."

That kind of gossip speeds from ear to lip. That was especially true in the small town I called home. The guys and I were talking about the steady date of a classmate of ours. Tank, one of my friends, almost spit when he said, "I thought Peter had more sense. If you're going to date girls, you have to have more self-control than that."

Those words roared back into my head nine months later when Tank, now home on his first Easter break from college, was saying, "I figure the only way I'll ever get married is if I have to." Back in those days "having to get married" meant "my girlfriend is pregnant and it's expected that I marry her."

What changed Tank? The influence of the people around him, the professors he respected, and the media he was reading or listening to. We Christians have a word for that. We'd say Tank was influenced by the world.

The World's Influence

The world does not agree that sexuality is a special gift from God. It doesn't see any reason for following God's guidelines for the use of our sexuality. The reason: the world looks at sexuality from a different vantage point. That makes its conclusions about sexuality much different.

It's like this. Look as closely at this page as your eyes will allow you to focus. If that were all you knew about this book, how would you describe it? Next hold the book at least an arm's length away. Would you describe the book differently now?

The way we view our sexuality can be like that little experiment. People can arrive at much different conclusions about their sexuality depending on the point from which they choose to look at it. People who don't know God's love in Jesus tend to see their sexuality up close. Christians can view their sexuality from a broader, more complete perspective.

The World's Conclusions about Sexuality

But often we Christians are influenced by the world's view of human sexuality, and we lose our perspective. "Everybody feels this way," we explain to ourselves, "I don't want to be weird." "Everybody's doing it" is just another variation.

Maybe you've been caught up in some of the world's philosophy on sex. Here are some of the conclusions the world has reached about sexuality. See if you know why they are wrong.

1. There Is No Difference between the Sexes

Some people would like us to believe that men and women are really not very different from one another and, if we would treat everyone like a human being rather than as a male or a female, many of the problems of the world would evaporate.

There are powerful authorities in our lives that say that. Some feminists tell women they must strive to compete in the male-dominated world of business by learning to practice the worst corporate strategies: underhanded grabbing for power, selfishness, and greed. Some rock stars add to the confusion with unisex dressing; it's hard to tell if they are male or female. Some television programs and movies would have us believe that men and women are interchangeable parts of a family. They show single parenting (or two "moms" and no dads or two "dads" and no moms) as just as good as having a father and mother.

Now it's certainly true that women have been denied many of the privileges men enjoy. Although women have matched and surpassed men in levels of higher education, they still earn less than men, and they don't make it as high on the corporate or political ladder.[1] That's not right. But neither is it right—perhaps the better word is honest—to say that there are only tiny differences between men and women.

Males and females are different. They are different in the obvious physical ways. They are also different in their emotional makeup, in the way they think, and in their attitudes. Women tend to make decisions based on intuition (how they feel about people, situations, or events). Men tend to rely on logic. But both intuition and logic are necessary for good decision making. Women tend to be more people oriented than men, caring more about others' needs and concerns. Men tend to be more task oriented than women, thinking it is more important to get a job done than to know how others feel while the job is getting done. Both perspectives are important. In fact, it's necessary for any organization, from families on up to multi-national conglomerates, to have leaders who are concerned about getting the job done and about the people who are part of the organization.

There are other differences. Males and females are influenced by different levels of hormones. The hormones females tend to have the most of promote gentleness, nurturing, and passivity. The hormones males tend to have the most of produce aggression, the need to be dominant, ambition, and sexual initiative. Every human being has both female and male hormones. The mixture of male and female hormones in each individual is unique, and that helps make each one of us different from everyone else in the world.

Please don't think, though, that because we are influenced by our hormones, we are slaves to their chemical commands. By God's power we can choose how we will act. We can't cop out of our personal responsibility to be sexually pure, even-tempered, or positive because "our hormones make us" sexually active, angry, or negative.

Obviously, God created males and females to complement one another, not to compete with each other. For our world, for any business, or for our families to function smoothly, we need both what women bring to those settings and what men bring. God has designed males and females with opposing characteristics so each will use his or her strengths to assist the other.

But then, that's the way God has made all of creation. Every part of nature is interdependent; one species depends on the other for support. (You've learned about food chains and symbiotic relationships in biology classes.) God has built his universe in a way that prevents one kind of organism from getting along all by itself. Rather, God's creation depends on all of its parts doing what they were designed to do while working in unselfish harmony.

2. There Are Lots of Differences Between the Sexes (Sexual Stereotypes)

Some people say there are no differences between men and women. Others say there are lots of differences and they tend to think of women as less capable than men. We call these assumed differences sexual stereotypes. A stereotype is the pattern we believe things of a certain type must fit. For example, believing that all girls are made of "sugar and spice and everything nice" and all boys are made of "toads and snails and puppy dog tails" is a stereotype. That stereotype assumes that every girl is sweet, kind, and gentle and every boy is ugly, low-down, and nasty.

There are many sexual stereotypes. Perhaps you believe a number of them. They include:

WOMEN aren't as smart as men,
make the best baby-sitters,
cry a lot,
are good cooks,
can't make good decisions,
like frilly clothes.

MEN are hunters and fishermen,
drink lots of alcohol,
are courageous,
earn the most in the family,
are the best leaders,
can't nurture children.

But God tells us, "You are all sons of God through faith in Christ Jesus, for all of you who were baptized into Christ have clothed yourselves with Christ. There is neither Jew nor Greek, slave nor free, male nor female, for you are all one in Christ Jesus" (Galatians 3:26-28).

Gender doesn't make any difference to God. Neither does race or social class. What does make a difference is Jesus. Since Jesus has made us God's sons, he has enabled us to inherit our Father's limitless wealth.

Does it strike you as sexist that God wants Christians to look at each other as his sons? When the New Testament was written, only sons could inherit from their fathers. So when God says "you are all sons of God through faith in Christ Jesus," he is telling us that Jesus has made every believer (male or female) a full inheritor of his grace. Whether male or female, we are all the same before God.

More than that, we are all fully gifted. 1 Peter 2:9 applies to every believer: "You are a chosen people, a royal priesthood, a holy nation, a people belonging to God, that you may declare the praises of him who called you out of darkness into his wonderful light." Whether male or female, we all enjoy the same high position: people chosen by God, royalty, priests, holy, God's prized possessions.

On the one hand, then, God wants us to see each other as equally important to him and to each other. On the other hand, he wants us to recognize that he has created us different from one another. Males are not better than females, nor are females better than males. We just serve different functions. Together we make a unit. Men and women need each other, because each supplies what the other doesn't have.

3. We Can Be Happy Only If Our Needs Are Being Met

"No, I don't want to."

When my daughters were preschoolers, I heard that a lot. "Eat your carrots." "No, I don't want to." "Come on along now, we're going shopping." "No, I don't want to." "It's time for bed. Hop on upstairs." "No, I don't want to."

Now don't laugh. You used to say that a lot yourself. So did I. When we're little, it's hard for us to see that there's good in anything that doesn't immediately make us happy. That shows our selfishness and immaturity.

The problem comes when people don't outgrow that attitude. People file for divorce because marriage doesn't allow them to do what they want to do. People ignore all the warnings and abuse drugs in order to meet their need to feel good at least for a short time. The world also warps our view of sexuality with "I don't want to" thinking. The world tells us it's fine to say "I don't want to" when we're told to save sex for the security of marriage. Sexuality, it tells us, should be used to make us happy—and however we choose to act sexually is OK as long as we are happy.

That's one of the reasons it's pretty much expected today that teenagers will be sexually active. Worse, it's assumed to be unthinkable to tell teens that sex before marriage will hurt them. After all, "We can be happy only if our needs are being met," and sexual intercourse satisfies our urges and makes us happy.

To the world, what the one who created sexuality says is unimportant. Some think the Bible's advice about being sexual beings is too old to apply to us modern people or too simple to make any sense to us sophisticated folks. Many people think it's better to listen to their desires than to their God.

Those of us who know how much our Creator loves us, however, strive to live by God's advice. "We love because he first loved us." He has washed all our sins away by punishing his Son in our place. What a marvelous gift! We're going to spend forever with him in heaven. And more: as long as we live on earth, he cares for us. By living in his world in a way which will please him, not us, we thank him for loving us.

4. We Must Be Free to Express Ourselves Sexually

Freedom is important to Americans. Our constitution guarantees us a number of wonderful freedoms including the freedom to practice our religion and the freedom to say and publish what we think. Sexual freedom is supposed to be one of our rights as well.

Unfortunately, the world's sexual freedom is not freedom at all. Here's why. You know how sin has messed up the way we think and act. (Remember what God said about humans: "From the time he is young, his thoughts are evil" Genesis 8:21 TEV.) Sin tells us good is bad and bad is good. It shouldn't surprise us then when people who aren't Christian tell us that there's nothing wrong with sex outside of marriage. It shouldn't even surprise us if sometimes Christians are misled and think that way. The sin within us doesn't permit us to see things as clearly as God sees them.

The effect of sin on our lives is like the effect of cocaine on an addict. For an addict, the highest good would seem to be the freedom to use all the cocaine he wants—even though we know that it's only the cocaine that is making him feel that way. He has become imprisoned by that drug. And the more he takes, the more imprisoned he is. So sin makes it seem to us that sexual activity with whomever we want, whenever we want, is real freedom. In reality, that's imprisonment.

God has created us to be like a train. A train is freest when it is running on its tracks. If a train should decide to jump its tracks because those tracks are too restrictive, how much freedom would that train gain? It would soon crash to a halt as its metal wheels would dig into the ground alongside the tracks.

Our sexuality is like that. As long as we are traveling down the tracks God has laid out for using our sexuality, we are free. The moment we jump those tracks for what we think is "freedom," we'll be bogged down, jammed up, and wrecked.

5. If It Feels Good, Do It

Playboy magazine has had quite an affect on our culture's sexual attitudes. "If it feels good, do it," is basically the Playboy philosophy. Another way of saying that is, "Whatever the pleasure, enjoy it. Don't let your personal hang-ups or anybody else's morality get in your way."

Unfortunately, for the same reasons we can't trust ourselves to know what real sexual freedom is, we can't trust ourselves to decide what pleasure is good for us or when it's good for us. Our basic sinfulness ruins our judgment. That's why we need to rely on God's word to tell us about the pleasures he's designed for us and how to use them.

Think about what happens when we believe pleasure is reason enough for doing whatever we do. That makes sex seem commonplace rather than a precious present from a loving Father. Worse, it makes pleasure into a god, for a god is whatever we value the most. And whatever we value the most will direct our actions. If pleasure is our god, we will live to get all the pleasure we can. That's why God says about immoral people, "Such a man is an idolater [and won't have] any inheritance in the kingdom of Christ and of God" (Ephesians 5:5).

On the other hand, the Scripture says, "In view of God's mercy (because he has loved you enough to punish his Son for your sins) . . . offer your bodies as living sacrifices, holy and pleasing to God—this is your spiritual act of worship" (Romans 12:1). Jesus is the reason we want to use God's gift of sex as he wants us to enjoy it.

6. Sex Is Healthy; Holding It Back Is Not

Some in our culture encourage the free use of sex because "it's healthy." What isn't healthy, they say, is repressing our sexual urges (not allowing our sex drive to express itself).

Christians certainly agree that sex is healthy for humans. We'd expect it to be good for us. It's a gift from God. Sex should be enjoyed. But at that point we part ways with the world. Christians maintain that we can be just as healthy with or without being sexually active.

Deciding not to act on our sexual urges is not sexual repression. Christians are not required to hinder the development of their sexuality. God requires only that we allow our sexuality to grow and bloom in the proper setting. Who would plant a flower seed in a flower pot that's stuck away in a dark closet? That plant would never amount to anything. Plants are designed by God to be out in the light. Sex outside of marriage keeps the beautiful plant of sex in the dark and incapable of ever fully blossoming. Marriage takes the plant of sex out of the closet and gives it light.

Christians may be accused of being ashamed of their sexuality, but there's no need for them to be ashamed. Our sexual nature, including our sex drive, is just as proper and wholesome as our body telling us it's hungry. Neither our urge for food nor the urge for sex is anything to be ashamed of. But Christians recognize a need to harness their sex drive, just as they harness their drive for food. If we ate every time our bodies told us they were a bit hungry, none of us would fit into compact cars. Giving in to our bodies whenever they tell us they crave sex will also deform us.

God has designed a time and place for sexual activity. It's called marriage. There sexual activity is healthy and can be fully enjoyed.

Some Guidelines

My friend Tank was influenced to change his views about the use of his sexuality by the people in his life. Whatever we allow to influence us will change our lives. That should tell us something about how to hang on to God's view of sexuality. If we are intent on using our gift of sexuality as God designed it, we need a lot of God's influence on our lives, and we need to minimize the world's influence.

Perhaps these guidelines will help you stay influenced by the right sources:

1. Stay tuned in to God's will for you. That's the only way you'll be able to tell when you are being swayed in the wrong direction. Constantly compare what people are telling you with what God is telling you. But notice: in order to make that comparison you have to know what God tells you. That means you can't get by without reading and studying God's word.

2. Watch whom you hang around with. The people we spend the most time with generally influence us the most. What kind of values do your friends have? We can also spend time with people by reading their writings. What kind of values do the authors of your magazines and books have? Proverbs 13:20 says, "He who walks with the wise grows wise, but a companion of fools suffers harm."

3. Remember that people who are not Christian look at life in a different way than you do. They don't know how much God loves them.

4. Remind yourself about God's love for you. "God so loved [you] that he gave his one and only Son, that [you] might. . . have eternal life" (John 3:16). Such a God could never ask you to do anything that wouldn't be good for you. That includes the way you are to use your sexuality.

5. Put God first. Jesus gave us a wonderful promise in Matthew 6:33: "Seek first his kingdom and his righteousness, and all these things [everything you need] will be given to you as well."

When God comes first in our lives, everything else

falls into place. And we want him to be first because of how deeply he's loved us, how completely he's forgiven us, and how well he cares for us. When we're taking time for Bible reading, prayer, worship, Scripture study with other believers, and the Lord's Supper, we are seeking his kingdom. Then we can expect him to keep his promise that "all these things will be given to you as well."

We can't expect that people who are not Christian will understand and support the way we feel about our sexuality and our commitment to enjoy sexual activity only within marriage. But because we know what our Father in heaven has done for us and the wonderful promises he keeps for us, we'll much rather do things his way than the way anyone else wants to do them.

It's so easy to get the wrong ideas about my sexuality, Jesus. It seems a lot of people around me are telling me things about sex that aren't true. Savior, I don't want to do the wrong things with any area of my life, and that includes how I use my sexuality. Keep me close to you so that I always know what is right and wrong and am strong enough to do the right thing and reject the wrong. Keep me reading and listening to your word so I find those insights and gain that power. Open my heart to believe what your word says. Then motivate me to do what you've told me. I want so badly to live in a way that makes you happy because you have guaranteed me a

place with you in heaven that will last forever—and because you take such good
care of me. Help me, Jesus.

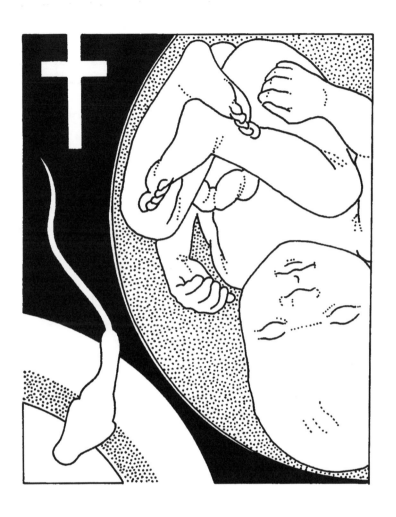

5.

ONCE UPON A TIME

"Once upon a time. . . ." Fairy tales start that way. Sometimes the story of how life begins is told to children like a fairy tale.

I remember being told that the stork brings babies and that my parents found me in the garden under a cabbage leaf. I wondered as a child whether being pregnant had anything to do with eating watermelon seeds. I recall being at a family gathering at the home of my grandparents when a younger cousin asked his mother what kind of food women needed to eat in order to have a baby. Choked laughs filled the room. My aunt turned red. Grandpa and Grandma turned grim-faced.

The conception and development of children, however, is far too miraculous and awe-inspiring to cloud with fairy tales. Here is the story of how you and I and everyone else all the way back to Cain began to be.

In the Beginning

Each one of us came to life in the darkness of our mother's Fallopian tube. In one of the Fallopian tubes a developed egg waits to be fertilized by a sperm, the male's contribution to conception. There are two Fallopian tubes. Each one links one of a woman's ovaries to the uterus or womb. Look at the diagram of the Fallopian tubes, ovaries, and uterus.

The sperm which reach the egg have tirelessly journeyed the four to five inches from the end of the vagina (called the cervix), into the uterus, and then up into the Fallopian tubes. Although those few inches do not seem far to us, when microscopic sperm are traveling that distance it's a long trip. Hundreds of millions of sperm begin the journey. Only the strongest ever reach the far-off egg, and then only one fertilizes it. Sometimes none are able to fertilize the egg. That, too, is part of God's plan. It helps insure a high percentage of physically healthy children.

A sperm has only one cell. But if you were to look at a sperm under a microscope, you would discover that it has three parts: a head, a neck, and a long tail. The tail moves back and forth to propel the sperm forward. The neck stores nutrition so the tail will have an energy source. The head is where 23 chromosomes are stored. When a sperm unites with an egg, those chromosomes pair with the 23 chromosomes of the egg and form a human being with 46 chromosomes.

It takes an electron microscope to see chromosomes, but if you could see them, you would notice they look a lot like strings. Attached to the strings are 15,000 genes. Each of those genes acts like a set of instructions to a fertilized egg, telling it the specifications to which it is to build that child. Genes establish the potential limits of one's size, intelligence, artistic abilities, and creativity. They also determine one's hair color, eye color, and likelihood of baldness. Every child will turn out different from every other because there are over 16 billion varying sets of instructions these genes are able to give. You would be a much different person today if God had used a different egg or different sperm to create you.

At the time fertilization takes place, the egg, which is about the size of a pinhead and many times the size of a sperm, is swarmed over by millions of sperm. Each sperm releases an enzyme which eats away at the egg's tough outer coating. (Notice again, God did not make fertilization easy. Only the strongest of the sperm will eventually enter the egg.) At last one sperm and only one will push its way inside. At that moment, the egg is fertilized and a new human being has been conceived. When that happens, the fertilized egg develops an even tougher coating, one the rest of the sperm cannot penetrate.

Twins

Twins can be conceived in one of two ways. Fraternal twins are conceived when two sperm cells each fertilize an egg. (It doesn't happen often, but sometimes both of a woman's ovaries produce a ripe egg at the same time.) Children from such a conception inherit different combinations of genes from their parents since every egg and every sperm have a different combination of genes. Fraternal twins may or may not be of the same sex. They look like any other brothers and sisters.

Identical twins, however, look exactly the same because they have the same combination of genes. Identical twins occur when a fertilized egg divides in two and the two halves become two different people. Since both come from the same fertilized egg, their genetic makeup is the same. Both have the same potential for developing their talents and abilities. However, because every human being has different experiences in life, is shaped by different people, and is influenced by different choices, even identical twins develop separate personalities, interests, and goals. God only makes people who are one of a kind.

The First Moments of Life

Within six to twelve hours after fertilization, the egg, now a one-celled human being, begins to divide. At first it divides and becomes two cells. Then those two cells become four cells and the process continues. At five days from conception, that tiny baby resembles an extremely small blackberry.

In the next days, that new life is pushed down the Fallopian tube into the uterus (womb) by tiny hairs which line those tubes. Once in the uterus, the fertilized egg attaches itself to the cushiony and nutrient-rich wall of the womb. The journey from the Fallopian tube to implantation in the uterus takes about a week.

A thin but tough bag then forms around the baby, and liquid accumulates inside. The liquid, called amniotic fluid, allows the baby to float peacefully and protects it from bumps and temperature changes. The amniotic fluid develops in the second week after conception.

When the baby attaches itself to the womb, another amazing development occurs. At the point of contact a placenta forms. The placenta is a wonderful organ which makes it possible for the baby to live in the womb. Its job is to filter out many harmful substances from a mother's blood while taking nourishment from her blood for the baby. The placenta also deposits wastes from the baby's blood into the mother's bloodstream so that her kidneys and liver can filter out those wastes and expel them through urination. The baby is attached to the placenta by an umbilical cord. The cord feeds into the baby at the navel.

It's also interesting to note that mother and child

have separate bloodstreams. Mother's and child's blood do not mingle. In fact, a child may have a completely different type of blood than her mother.

Signs of Life

Somewhere between the 18th and 25th day from conception the baby's tiny heart begins to beat. Brain waves have been recorded as early as after 40 days. They are definitely present by eight weeks (56 days). Four weeks from conception a baby is about the size of an apple seed. At eight weeks a baby responds to touch; its eyes, ears and nose are taking shape. Actually, all the baby's body systems are present by the eighth week (they will be working by week eleven), and the baby definitely looks like a tiny human being. For example, if you were to see the baby, you could easily tell whether it was male or female. (By the way, almost all abortions are done on pre-born children who are eight to ten weeks old.)

By week eleven or twelve the baby begins to breathe. Since there is no air in the amniotic sac, he breathes in the amniotic fluid. He will do this steadily until birth. He doesn't drown because oxygen is supplied him from his mother through his umbilical cord. By week eighteen his vocal chords are developed enough so that he could cry if he could breathe air.

Since the child depends on its mother for oxygen, it is harmed if the mother smokes. Smoking robs blood of oxygen and consequently deprives the pre-born. In some cases smoking mothers have caused their children to be malnourished and even brain damaged.

After Three Months

Before the end of the third month (eleven to twelve weeks) the baby has fingernails and weighs about an ounce. By the end of the next month he will weigh six ounces, and at the end of the fifth month he will weigh a pound. It is at this weight that a mother begins to feel the baby moving around. On the day a mother first feels the movements of her baby, the child is said to be quickened, which means made alive. Many years ago, it was falsely thought babies were not living until quickening happened.

By this time in a child's life its nostrils, ears, and eyes are functioning. It can hear sounds from outside the womb and quickly learns to recognize its mother's voice. It can see light coming into the womb through its mother's skin.

Pre-born children are quite aware of their surroundings. That makes it important that they be given a loving, gentle stay in the womb. Children can be frightened during their time in the womb. Tim La Haye in his book *Sex Education Is for the Family* reports:

I am familiar with one case in which a child began crying within minutes after birth when she heard her father's voice. As the parents were interviewed, they admitted that they had had some furious arguments during the pregnancy. This unfortunate child came into the world afraid of her own father, learning to fear his voice while she was still inside her mother's womb (page 25).

The Final Months

During the final months of pregnancy the child continues to grow rapidly. From one pound at five months, it will weigh five to eight pounds (or more) at birth four months later. (What would you have to do in order to weigh five times your weight four months from now?)

Doctors and scientists have a variety of names to describe the stages of a pre-born baby's life. At first a pre-born is called a fertilized ovum (egg). It is called a zygote when it attaches to the wall of the uterus and a blastocyst following that point. For the remainder of the first eight weeks, the baby is called an embryo. From week eight on, it is called a fetus (Latin for baby).

Prenatal Checkups

It is essential that expectant mothers begin a routine of regular checkups with an obstetrician (OB/GYN) or family physician. A doctor will monitor both the mother's and the baby's health throughout the pregnancy. A physician can find any irregularities in the pregnancy and take appropriate steps to remedy them. Christian mothers will want to research the background of their doctor and be sure to ask whether he/she is pro-life. It seems to me that a doctor who is also in the business of killing pre-born babies would find it hard to be dedicated to helping other pre-born babies through their first months.

Birth Defects

Most pre-born children who are not developing

properly die before birth. For example, sometimes internal organs do not form as they should. As the child grows and those organs do not begin functioning, the child dies, just as you would die if your heart or lungs or liver stopped working.

When a baby dies from natural causes before it is born, we call that a miscarriage. Just as people die when they are 96 years old and 36 years old and 6 years old and 6 days old, so people can die when they are moments from conception, days from conception, or months from conception.

Other defects may be caused by genetic combinations that don't work right. When that happens, the baby doesn't develop properly. Most such babies die before birth, usually in the first three months.

Circumstances in the lives of mothers can cause birth defects in their children. Some mothers harm their pre-born children by poor eating habits, drinking alcohol, and using drugs. Mothers with addiction to heroin pass their addiction on to their children. Expectant mothers should not have x-rays taken, especially in the early weeks of pregnancy. Expectant mothers who have contracted rubella (German measles) may also give birth to defective children. Women who become pregnant prior to their eighteenth birthday or after their fortieth birthday also run a higher than average risk of giving birth to a child with defects.

When mothers have a negative blood type (like O-) and fathers have a positive blood type (like A+), there will be a risk to the life of the second child they have. This is called having an Rh-negative factor. The second child is in danger because of the way the mother's body reacts at the birth of the first child. At the birth of the first child, the mother's blood begins to produce anti-bodies because of the conflicting blood types. Actually the mother's body is fooled into thinking the first baby was a disease that had to be fought off. (Antibodies in the blood protect a body from germs. Antibodies are also at work when transplanted organs are rejected.) When another child is conceived, the mother's body is now on alert, armed and ready to fight against that baby's presence. The second and all other children can be spared harm if the mother has a special vaccination after her first child is born or miscarried.

Many procedures can help children with abnormali-ties. Doctors are developing new ways to correct defects before a child's birth. That's why mothers should be sure to have prenatal checkups, especially if they are in their teens or beyond the later thirties.

Premature Births

Children who are born before they have spent nine months (40 weeks) in the womb are called premature. In recent years medical science has made fantastic strides in saving the lives of premature children. Many children who are born after just 20 weeks in the womb are now being rescued from what used to be certain death. These children may weigh only about a pound and have severe breathing problems. Nonethe-less, doctors expect that in the future even younger children will be saved.

Gender Determination

The sperm determines which gender a baby will be.

A mother's egg has just one set of chromosomes. Doctors call them X chromosomes. Sperm come in two kinds, X and Y. If an X sperm fertilizes the egg, the baby will be a female, a Y sperm will produce a male.

Infertility

When couples are not able to have children, that is called infertility. The way God designed the human body to start and nurture new life is extremely complex. Something wrong with just one part of the reproductive system can stop a new human being from being conceived or from developing properly. Medicine has learned how to help many childless couples. A married couple that is experiencing problems in conceiving children should talk with a doctor.

In spite of advances in medicine, however, some couples will never be able to have children. This can be difficult for them to accept. So it is important, especially when the sadness about not being able to have children is fresh, for a couple to remind themselves about God's love for them (in order to provide forgiveness for us, he didn't even hold back his own Son) and God's plan for their lives that's built on that love.

Childbirth

No one has been able to figure out how a mother's body knows when it's time to give birth. But about a week before a child is born it usually turns head down in the womb and settles into the pelvic cavity. Doctors refer to this as the baby's dropping.

The discomfort a mother goes through before childbirth is called labor. Labor begins with mild cramps, which often feel like menstrual cramps. They last about 30 seconds and come 15-20 minutes apart. Then the cramps gradually become closer together and increase in intensity. When the time between the cramps is under ten minutes, couples usually go to the hospital.

At some point during labor the amniotic sac is likely to break, and the fluid drains off. It flushes out of the birth canal and is eliminated. This is referred to as a mother's "water breaking." Doctors advise mothers to come to the hospital immediately when their water breaks even if contractions are still far apart. Without the amniotic fluid to protect it, the baby can easily be hurt.

During labor, the cervix, which has tightly sealed the womb from the vagina for nine months, expands to about four inches wide so that the baby might pass down the birth canal and out of the mother's body. The uterus, the largest and most powerful muscle in a woman's body, pushes the baby downward as it contracts. Toward the end of labor, the mother uses her abdominal muscles to help with the pushing.

Normally, the baby's head appears first, then its shoulders. After that the child is quickly freed from the birth canal. The baby is still attached to the umbilical cord and the placenta. The placenta or afterbirth is expelled from the womb shortly after the baby is born. Nurses suction any mucus from the child's mouth and nose, and the baby is encouraged to breathe on its own if it is not already doing so.

Usually the child is quickly cleaned and presented to the parents. In many delivery rooms the parents are immediately allowed to hold their child. Sometimes the father is permitted to cut the umbilical cord. The cord is cut about three inches from the navel. In a few days it will dry up and fall off.

The entire birth process may take from eight to twenty hours. Usually the first child's birth requires more time than subsequent births. There is pain involved in giving birth, but women who have learned about the childbirth process tend to experience less pain than those who know little about giving birth. Mothers can also learn special exercises and techniques for breathing that will ease the discomfort of labor.

Parents often attend childbirth classes to prepare themselves for this time. These classes make childbirth a safer experience for mother and child. They also help mothers to know what to expect, and they assist fathers in becoming part of the birthing team.

It's No Fairy Tale

God's plan for the first nine months of our lives is no fairy tale. It's an amazing phenomenon that God allows parents to participate in. The psalmist certainly had it right when he wrote:

You created my inmost being: you knit me together in my mother's womb. I praise you because I am fearfully and wonderfully made; your works are wonderful, I know that full well. My frame was not hidden from you when I was made in the secret place. When I was woven together in the depths of the earth, your eyes saw my unformed body. All the days ordained for me were written in your book before one of them came to be. How precious to me are your thoughts, O God! How vast is the sum of them! (Psalm 139:13-17)

Now is probably a great time to thank God for creating you with just the right set of chromosomes from your mother and father so you could be the unique and valuable person you are.[2]

O God, the Creator of all life, you made me in a way that urges me to stand in awe of you. You took me from a tiny, single cell with just the right chromosomes and built me into the person I am today. And you keep on working on me—shaping, honing, improving me—so that I might serve you in just the way you want me to serve. It's fantastic to think that I am here for a reason: that you have created me for this time in the world's history to accomplish something no one else could ever do. Help me to sense your leadership in my life so I always strive to live out your will. I want that for my life because you have not only created me and preserved my life; you have forgiven me and provided me with eternal life through Jesus.

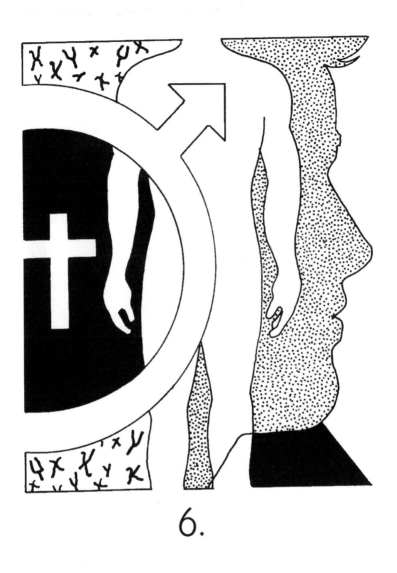

6.

THE MALE HALF OF THE REPRODUCTIVE SYSTEM

MALE GENITALIA – SIDE VIEW

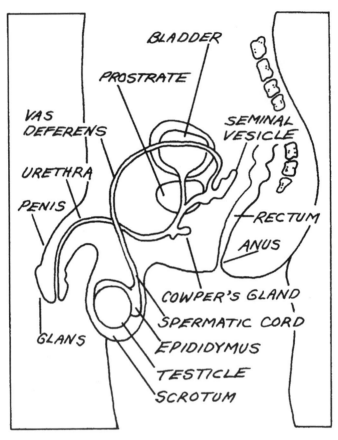

"Momma! Momma!" My four-year-old niece yanked at her mother's arm. Her eyes were wide. She had just made a shocking discovery. She and her male cousin, who was also four, had just come from the bathroom.

"Momma! Momma!" she gasped, "Freddie goes tinkle from his belly button!"

Granted, she didn't have it quite right, but my niece had uncovered a startling truth. Boys and girls aren't built the same under their clothes. And for good reason. Their genitals serve different purposes.

There are obvious differences between the appearance of the genitals of males and females. Most of the male reproductive organs are located outside the body where they can be seen. Most of the female reproductive organs are tucked away inside the body.

We're going to take a look at the female reproductive system in the next chapter. In this chapter we'll talk about the male's reproductive organs.[3]

Sperm and Testicles

Sperm is the most important contribution the male makes to human reproduction. Sperm is produced in the testicles (testicles are also called the testes). The testicles are oblong glands about the size of a large marble, which hang in a sack called the scrotum. The testes are attached to the body by spermatic cords. The left testicle hangs down slightly lower than the right in order to prevent damage from the two testicles bumping together. One testicle is slightly larger than the other.

The scrotum has a separate compartment for each testicle and is secured to the body at the base of the penis. Depending on the temperature, the scrotum may allow the testes to hang down and away from the body or pull them up close to the body. The reason is that the testicles can produce sperm only if they are four degrees cooler than the body. The action of the muscles in the scrotum helps maintain that cooler temperature.

From the time puberty begins (in males, when their body starts producing sperm), the testicles manufacture hundreds of millions of sperm each day. Sperm production continues throughout the life of each male. Men cannot use up all their sperm by having sex too often. Nor can men harm themselves by having sex a number of times in a row. A male's reproductive machinery will function repeatedly for several times in quick succession (especially if the male is young). But there will come a point when the body will not be able to repeat the sex act. After a period of rest, the reproductive system will be able to function again.

The sperm are so tiny that one drop can contain 120 million. Under a microscope sperm look like tiny tadpoles. The testicles also produce an important hormone called testosterone. This hormone controls the development of male sex characteristics like facial hair and a lower voice. It also brings about rapid growth of muscles and bones during puberty.

If the testicles do not function properly, the male is not able to impregnate his spouse even though he is able to experience orgasm. (Orgasm is the feeling of pleasure that occurs for males when sperm are released from the penis.) Sometimes a man's testicles produce just a few sperm. Since it takes only one sperm to fertilize a female's egg, causing a pregnancy is still possible even if the man's sperm count is low. However, the chances of fertilization taking place are reduced considerably. If a man loses his testicles through an accident or surgery, he will no longer be able to impregnate his wife. The loss of one testicle, however, will not make him infertile.

Each testicle contains a long, but tiny tube. Each tube measures about 1000 feet in length. It is in these tubes that the sperm are produced. From these tiny tubes the sperm move on to the larger tubes which connect the testes to the body (the epididymis). The epididymis serves as an incubator and storage area where the sperm mature. From there the sperm travel inside the body through a canal called the vas deferens to the seminal vesicles for continued storage. The sperm are kept here until needed. The seminal vesicles are located in two pouches just behind the bladder.

Next to the seminal vesicles is another important reproductive gland called the prostate. This gland constantly produces a fluid which is mixed with fluid from other glands to form semen. Semen is a whitish, sticky liquid within which the sperm leave the penis during ejaculation. (Ejaculation happens at orgasm when sperm are forced from the penis in several rapid-fire bursts.) The semen provides the sperm with a liquid to swim in as they attempt to make their way to a female's egg. The prostate gland also assists in ejaculation by contracting and pushing the sperm out.

The Cowper's gland serves an important function in reproduction, as well. The fluid this gland releases when a male becomes sexually excited neutralizes and flushes away any urine left in the urethra (the tube through which the urine leaves the body). Without this fluid the acidity of the urine would kill the sperm.

Penis

The penis hangs directly in front of the scrotum. It is designed to fulfill two purposes. It is the canal for urine on its way out of the body. It also allows a male to deposit his sperm several inches inside the body of his sex partner near the opening to the cervix and as close as possible to her ripened egg. A valve at the base of the penis makes it impossible for urination and ejaculation to take place at the same time.

Ejaculation occurs after the penis has been stimulated by rubbing and is erect. During that process semen moves into the urethra and at the moment of orgasm strong muscles propel the semen out of the penis.

At the tip of the penis is the glans. The densely packed nerve endings which it contains make the glans especially sensitive to touch. During intercourse, the rubbing of the glans inside the vagina provides the male with the most physical pleasure of any touching experience.

At birth the glans is covered with a skin jacket, often called a foreskin. Usually the foreskin is removed by a simple surgical procedure when the baby is a day or two old. This is called circumcision. The foreskin provides some additional protection for the glans, but it is not necessary for enhancing reproduction or sexual stimulation. Circumcision is generally performed to assist males in keeping that part of their body clean since a foreskin will trap dirt and urine next to the glans. Circumcised males also seem to lower the incidence of cervical cancer for their wives.

Erection

In order for sexual intercourse to take place, the penis must become erect. Normally the penis measures three to four inches at rest. It may be smaller. At rest it is soft and pliable. When sexually stimulated, however, the penis stretches to about six inches, swells in circumference, and becomes firm enough to lift itself upward and stand away from the body. In erection the penis has a slight outward curve, which matches the curve of the vagina.

During early puberty higher hormone levels encourage more frequent erections. Erections may happen as a result of sexually stimulating thoughts. They may occur for no apparent reason. They may occur almost anywhere: at dances, during movies, at school, or because of tight jeans. An erection will go away if it is ignored.

At times adolescent boys feel embarrassed because of these erections. However, they are a normal part of growing up and should be viewed as the body's readying itself for marriage.

Involuntary erections will occur during a male's lifetime. Often men awaken with an erection. This is due to higher hormone levels in their blood. Erections also will occur several times during sleep even though the male will not be experiencing any sexually stimulating dreams. (Be sure to read the section on wet dreams in chapter ten.)

Some young men worry whether the size of their penis will be large enough or perhaps too large to give pleasure to their wives. God has created women to receive sexual stimulation at the outer edge of the vagina rather than deep within. Penis length will not increase a woman's sexual stimulation. Also keep in mind that the vagina is a flexible tube which is able to expand sufficiently to permit a baby to pass through.

It will certainly be flexible enough to accommodate a penis of any size.

Pain or Swelling

There may be times when a male is stimulated almost to orgasm but then—for whatever the reason—the stimulation stops. This usually results in some discomfort for the male, a dull ache in his groin. Street slang calls this condition "blue balls." This condition is not harmful and will pass in several minutes. It is not necessary for a male in this situation to have an orgasm, even though men have sometimes lied and used that as a way to get their dates to have sex with them. It's not true when men say to their girlfriends, "If we don't go all the way now, you'll hurt me."

When males are hit in the scrotum, severe pain can result. To avoid injury to these organs when playing in athletic contests where there will be rough-housing, men should wear an athletic supporter. They should also consider wearing a metal or plastic protector which is inserted into an athletic supporter. It fits in front of and around the penis and scrotum. Most pharmacies carry these items.

If a male experiences prolonged pain in his scrotum or if swelling occurs, he should go to a doctor. Sometimes the cord attached to a testicle will twist and cause blood to back up in the testicle. If this is not corrected, the testicle may be damaged enough to stop producing sperm. A doctor can easily diagnose this and correct it if necessary.

Men sometimes have to deal with a fungus related to athlete's foot which grows in their groin. Often this is called "jock itch." This fungus causes the skin on the scrotum and the inside of the thighs to be red and sore. Any pharmacy has effective medicines to cure this condition.

We're Not Built the Same

God has built men with a reproductive system that's astounding. If you are a male, you've got a lot to thank God for—especially when it comes to the genitals God has given you. Far from being a part of your body to be ashamed of and to poke fun of, your reproductive organs should lead you to thank God for being so wise. Girls and boys are different, as my little niece discovered. Our genitals aren't the same. In the next chapter we'll discover how girls are different from boys—and how even more wonderful the God who made us really is.

Dear heavenly Father, in your wisdom you have made males and females to be very similar, but also very different. Thank you for making males as you have. The wonderful way you have designed their part of the human reproductive system is really something. I know now that those special organs are not to be made fun of, because they are one of your loving gifts to men. And I don't have to feel ashamed when I learn about those parts or talk about them. They are part of your wonderful miracle of creation. So thank you, Lord, for making men as you have. You are a fantastic God!

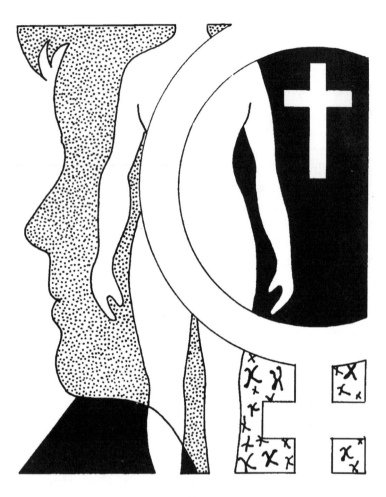

7.

THE FEMALE HALF OF THE REPRODUCTIVE SYSTEM

FEMALE GENITALIA — SIDE VIEW

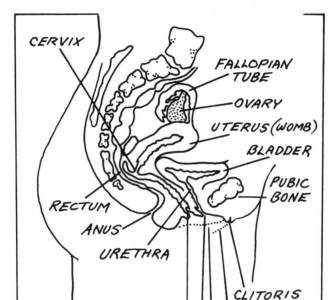

CERVIX
FALLOPIAN TUBE
OVARY
UTERUS (WOMB)
BLADDER
PUBIC BONE
RECTUM
ANUS
URETHRA
CLITORIS
LABIA MAJORA
LABIA MINORA
MEATUS
HYMEN
VULVA

The way God designed the male reproductive system to work is a marvel, but the female reproductive system is even more astounding. It is there that the Lord of continuing creation calls human life into existence, nurtures it, nourishes it, hugs it in the womb's loving arms, and then sends it out into our world to accomplish his purposes.

What we can say about the female half of the

human reproductive system can't possibly do justice to the wonderful way God has created women to nurture new life. Don't allow the clinical terms to detract from the wonderful ways God works through the female reproductive system. And, if you are a female, don't forget to praise him for making you in such an astounding way.[4]

Internal Organs

The female reproductive system consists of the external and the internal organs. The internal organs begin with the ovaries. The ovaries, about the size and shape of almonds, are located just below the hip bones.

Each ovary contains about 400,000 undeveloped eggs. (God wanted to make sure that women would be equipped to bear children!) Only about 300-400 of these eggs ripen during a woman's years of fertility. Sometime between the ages of 10 and 12 the ovaries begin to produce the hormone estrogen. Similar to the male hormone testosterone, this hormone starts a female body toward puberty. The ovaries also produce another female hormone called progesterone. The ovaries will continue to manufacture these hormones until menopause (the time in a woman's life when her body stops producing eggs).

From the beginning of puberty the ovaries ripen an egg about every 28 days. The ripened egg bursts from the ovaries and is caught in the Fallopian tube which hovers over each ovary. From there the egg or ovum is carried along further by fluids and tiny hairs into the tube. The egg stays in the tube two to three days awaiting fertilization by a sperm.

If the egg happens to be fertilized, it continues its journey into the uterus and attaches itself to the wall of the uterus, and a new human being's nine months in the womb begin.

The uterus is an upside-down pear-shaped organ, about four inches long in a mature woman. It has been wonderfully designed to house a child during pregnancy. Its walls are made of extremely elastic muscle, the largest and most powerful muscle in a woman's body. It is contractions of this muscle that cause cramps during menstruation.

Between the uterus and the vagina is another muscle, the cervix, which holds the end of the uterus shut, allowing only the monthly menstrual flow and sperm to pass through. During pregnancy the cervix, sealed with a mucus plug, holds the child in the womb. It expands during labor, however, to allow the child to be born.

The vagina, also called the birth canal, like the uterus is made of elastic muscles. It is three to five inches long. Most of the time the walls of the vagina touch each other, similar to a deflated balloon. As mentioned in the last chapter, the vagina will expand to accept a penis of any size. During sexual intercourse, the vagina produces a lubricating fluid which makes the sex act more pleasurable. In some women, additional fluid will be secreted at the moment of orgasm.

The vagina cleans itself by secreting another type of fluid called leucorrhea. This whitish fluid washes the vagina and is then expelled. It is present in varying amounts during any month. Some women wear thin sanitary napkins to soak up the leucorrhea. If the leucorrhea ever takes on a dark yellowish color or if it causes itching and burning, a physician should be consulted. Those symptoms may indicate a bladder or vaginal infection.

Douches have been gaining popularity among American women. A douche cleanses the vagina by squirting water along with some kind of gentle cleanser up into the vagina. Even though advertising has made douching acceptable and a number of companies are making lots of money by selling douches, it is not necessary. God has designed the female body to cleanse itself. Women do well not to be tricked by Madison Avenue into buying something they don't need.

External Organs

A woman's external sexual organs are called the vulva. Pubic hair is considered part of the vulva. The purpose of this hair is to protect the area from irritation and perspiration. Men also find the sight of pubic hair stimulating.

The hymen is a thin membrane that partly covers the opening to the vagina. It is found only in humans. A woman's virginity used to be determined by the condition of her hymen. It was thought that the hymen could be broken only through sexual intercourse. Because of that, in years gone by, if the hymen was intact on a woman's wedding night, that was accepted as proof that she was a virgin. However, we know today that the state of a hymen is not a good indicator of a woman's virginity. The hymen can be torn by any number of activities, including athletics and the use of tampons. Still other hymens are not torn even after sexual relations.

The opening to the vagina is surrounded by two cushiony folds of skin which resemble lips. The outer set of lips are called the labia majora (the major lips), and the inner set are called the labia minora (the minor lips). The outer side of the labia majora are covered with pubic hair and serve to protect the genital area. The labia minora add further protection to the vagina. In some women the inner lips are completely hidden by the outer lips. In others the inner lips stick out beyond the outer lips. The lips may be pink to brown in color; they may be wrinkled or smooth. God has made everyone unique, and none of these variations is cause for concern.

The clitoris is a raised area of skin at the top of the labia minora. Usually about pea-sized, it can be larger. Its function is similar to the male's glans. The clitoris is rich in nerve endings, which makes it highly sensitive to touch.

The urethra opens from the body at a point about half way between the clitoris and the vagina. This small opening is called the meatus. Urine leaves the body from this opening. Unlike the penis, which serves as the channel for urine and semen, the female body has completely separate openings for urination and sexual relations.

Breasts

Although a woman's breasts are not really a part of her reproductive system, God has designed them to feed the baby she gives birth to. After a baby is born, a mother's breasts begin to produce special milk. This milk provides a baby with nourishment tailored just for human babies and with protection from some kinds of sicknesses. Mothers who breast-feed their babies also promote a close emotional bond between themselves and their children. It is a pleasurable experience for both the mother and the baby. Mother's milk can nourish a newborn for many months.

During puberty the breasts, or mammary glands, grow and develop. The size and shape of a woman's breasts are determined mostly as a result of her genes. Just as some girls are taller or shorter than others, some girls have larger or smaller breasts than others. The size of breasts makes no difference in a mother's ability to feed her children. Nor are women with larger breasts more stimulated during sexual intercourse. Breasts are the size they are because of the amount of fatty tissue they contain.

Sometimes girls worry because their breasts are not both the same size. Breasts develop at different rates during puberty, and even when they are fully developed, breasts may not be the same size.

There's More

We've got more to say about the awesome way God has designed a woman's reproductive organs. In the next chapter we'll talk about how the Lord prepares a woman's body for the possibility of starting and sheltering a new life.

Lord God, you do the most wonderful things. The way you have designed human females so they are able to hold, nurture, and protect the newest of life within their wombs is terrific. Thank you for making

women the way you have and for enabling girls to grow into women. It makes me feel so secure and loved knowing that you have that all worked out. Knowing these things adds to my feelings of security and of love that I've found in Jesus, who guarantees me I am right with you. Thanks.

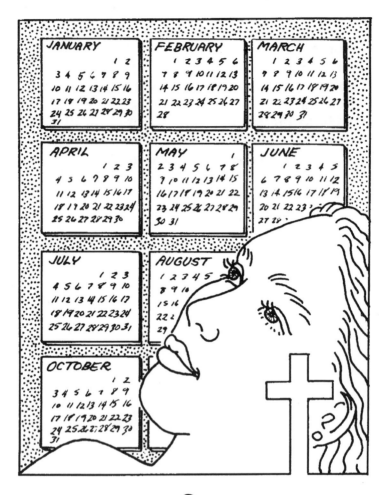

8.

Monthly Preparations
for New Life

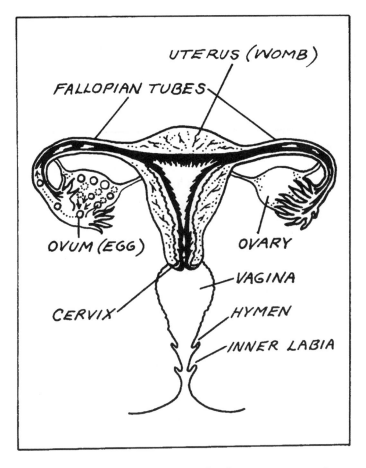

Something like a miracle happens within a woman's body each month. Sometimes women think of it more as a bother, but it's still an astounding wonder made possible by a loving and wise God.

Readying for New Life

Once about every 28 days a woman's pituitary gland, which is attached to the base of the brain, signals one of the ovaries to ripen one egg. This mature egg, then, bursts forth from the ovary and is caught by the end of the Fallopian tube that is positioned over that ovary. The egg makes its way down into that Fallopian tube. There it waits for the opportunity to be fertilized and to become a human being.

During this time the woman's body has been busily making other preparations, should fertilization happen. The uterus, urged on by the estrogen and progesterone hormones produced in the ovaries, has clothed itself with extra blood vessels. If the egg waiting in the Fallopian tube is fertilized, that new human life will be carried on down out of the tube and into the uterus. There it will seek to cling to the soft, blood-vessel-rich uterine wall. Once attached, it will continue growing into a baby that will be able to live in the outside world. During this time of the month the woman's body waits expectantly, poised to set the machinery in motion, should conception occur.

Usually the egg is not fertilized. Each time that happens, the egg is expelled from the Fallopian tubes into the uterus, and the uterus shakes off its soft lining since it is no longer necessary. The time of the month when a woman's body discards the unfertilized egg and the special lining of the uterus is called menstruation.

Menstruation

Menstruation, or a woman's monthly period, has been thought by some to be a curse. But how wrong that is. Menstruation is a wonderful blessing. It is regular proof that a woman has within her the capacity to bear children, to give life to another human being.

These monthly cycles begin as early as age nine in some girls. Most girls have their first period about age thirteen; some not until age sixteen. Any of those ages is normal. The beginning of menstruation is called menarche (men-ar-key), which also marks the start of puberty. In some societies menarche is a cause for great celebration—another girl has become capable of bearing children. It should be a time of celebration for us, as well!

At first the menstrual cycles may be irregular. Some cycles may run long, others short. Sometimes months will be skipped altogether. A number of months after menarche, however, the cycles will settle into a pattern of around 28 days. Some women's cycles are as short as 20 days; others have up to 35-day cycles. The menstruation period lasts from three to seven days.

It may happen that a period comes early or late. Worry, stress, illness, excitement, or severe dieting can be the cause. Women who are in strict physical conditioning programs have found that their menstrual cycles completely shut down. A regular routine, a normal diet, and adequate sleep will help maintain a fairly constant menstrual cycle. If a teenage girl's period is not regular after a year from menarche, she should mention this to her physician.

Menstrual cycles continue until a woman's ovaries quit producing eggs. This is called menopause, and it takes place during a woman's forties or fifties.

Menstruation lasts from three to five days. During that time a woman loses from a quarter to a half cup of blood. It is a completely normal part of being a human. Menstruation is a sign of a healthy body. It is nothing for a woman to be embarrassed about and certainly nothing to be ashamed of.

Menstrual Discomfort

It is not unusual for women to feel some discomfort during their period. Menstrual cramps may be felt in the lower abdomen. This should not stop women from carrying on their regular activities, however. During this time of the month, women do well to avoid becoming chilled, to exercise moderately rather than strenuously, to steer clear of rich foods, to get enough sleep, and to drink plenty of water.

For some women there is a slight weight gain during their period. This is because their bodies hold more fluids. This lasts for only a few days. Women may also experience bad moods and higher than normal feelings of tension during menstruation. This, too, is temporary and will stop once the period comes to an end. Soreness in the breasts often alerts women to the beginning of menstruation. This is normal.

It is not unusual that the flow of blood will be heavier on one day than on another. The color of the flow may range from bright red to rusty brown.

Sometimes when menarche begins, girls feel embarrassed. They may think that "everybody knows" they are having their period. They may worry about odor. They may be afraid that classmates will tease them. These are normal emotions. As girls get older, they become more comfortable with the monthly cycle God has built into their body's clock, and those fears go away. If you know someone who is embarrassed about menstruation, you might suggest they seek advice from a woman they trust and feel comfortable around.

Premenstrual Syndrome (PMS)

A small percentage of women (doctors estimate 5%) have more severe pre-menstrual symptoms. They may suffer headaches painful enough to disrupt their ability to function normally. They may experience a dull abdominal ache, tenderness in their breasts, and a feeling of fullness. This has been named premenstrual syndrome (PMS).

Doctors are able to treat this syndrome, but on an individual basis. A woman should never be satisfied with a treatment that is not tailored to her PMS symptoms. Physicians can treat PMS by correcting hormonal balances and prescribing other drugs.

Women with more than normal discomfort connected with menstruation have found that they can help the situation by cutting down on salt, sugar, and caffeine during the week before menstruation. Additional doses of vitamin B, eating a balanced diet, and herbal diuretics also are of assistance. If pursued for several months, daily exercise will also give relief. Lessening tension in one's life is also beneficial.

Menstrual Myths

Through the years a number of myths about menstruation have arisen. One myth says that menstruation is an illness. It is not. It is a normal part of every healthy woman's life. It is a cause of rejoicing, because the monthly period testifies to that woman's ability to produce new life.

Some have said that menstruation is a curse God has placed on women. God's pronounced punishment on Eve in Genesis 3:16 ("with pain you will give birth to children") is supposed to mention that curse. However, God had previously "blessed" Eve and told her to "be fruitful and increase in number" [Genesis 1:28]. Part of that blessing was granting her body the privilege of preparing an egg for fertilization each month and, if the egg was not fertilized, to wash it away [menstruation]. The menstrual cycle is a blessing from God.

Another myth is that menstruation is cause for stopping women from handling more responsible jobs. There are people who believe that women can't handle responsibility well because once a month a woman's energy levels and mood will change. That, however, is no reason to deny women responsible positions. Menstruation normally causes only minor discomfort and will not affect the ability of a woman to do her job.

Some people believe that the cramps which sometimes accompany menstruation are not real. This is not true. The cramps are caused when the uterus, the largest and most powerful muscle in a woman's body, contracts as it sheds that special layer of blood vessels it had built up for a possible baby to live on.

That menstruation is dirty is another myth. Perhaps this myth sprang from the odor which sometimes accompanies menstruation. The odor is not from the bloody discharge, however. Odor happens when that discharge is allowed to interact with warmth and air. The odor can be eliminated when pads and tampons are changed regularly and the woman keeps herself clean. At times tampons and pads will have to be changed several times during the day and during the night. Most women have to make that change at least every four hours. Because they allow the flow to come into contact with the air, pads will have to be changed more frequently than tampons if odor is to be avoided.

Absorbing the Flow

Sanitary napkins or pads are preferred by some women. They work well except when swimming. They come with adhesive strips on the back and stick to one's underpants. Napkins come in various levels of absorbency to match the amount of menstrual flow (for example, maxi-pads and mini-pads).

Many women have found that tampons are the most convenient way to absorb the menstrual flow. Tampons are soft absorbent cylinders which are inserted into the vagina. Girls who have never used tampons before may wish to ask their mothers for advice before using them.

When inserting a tampon for the first time, the important thing to remember is to relax. Next, find a time when you will not be bothered. Separate the folds of the labia to find the opening to the vagina. Gently push the tampon inside. It should completely disappear beyond the muscles at the opening of the vagina. You can be assured that it will not go too far and that it will not fall out.

When a tampon is used the first time, nervousness may cause the muscle at the opening to the vagina to tighten up, so take your time. The hymen may also make it hard to insert the tampon. Directions for using tampons are printed on every box.

To dispose of a pad, fold it in half, wrap toilet paper around it, and put it in the waste container in your bathroom. Never place it in the toilet. Most of the time, used tampons can be flushed down the toilet, but check with your parents first. Tampons have been known to clog some toilets. Some brands of sanitary protection come individually wrapped. Those wrappings and any applicators should always be disposed of in a wastebasket, never in a toilet.

A Special Gift

Menstruation is a reminder of the special gift God has granted women: the gift of nurturing new life within their bodies. When menstruation stops, that gift is lost. Remember to thank God for his gift to you whenever it's "that time of the month."

The way you create life in the womb and help it grow and develop is astounding, my dear Father. And to think that I was once alive in my mother's womb. Each month you ready a woman's body for nourishing a new life. Menstruation is the evidence of a woman's ability to be part of that wonder. Thank you for that wonderful reminder to women of the great privilege you have given them. Thank you, too, for the miracle of eternal life you have shown us through your Son. I pray this prayer through faith in him.

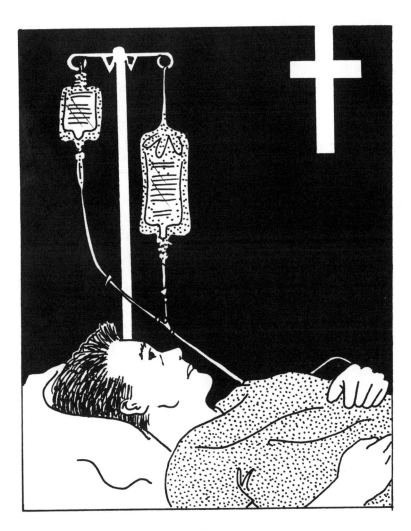

9.

It Can Make You Sick

Al Capone died from it. Capone was a Chicagoland gangster of Prohibition days, but his memory was still very much alive when I was growing up. Capone died in prison of a venereal disease he had caught years before; syphilis, as I recall. I was told it was a horrible death, coming after the disease had eaten its way into his brain.

The warnings I was given about pre-marital sexual activity took on a whole new meaning in junior high when I learned about venereal disease (VD). I was especially concerned after I listened to (untrue) stories about people catching VD from toilet seats.

Back then the only two sexually transmitted diseases (STDs) people talked much about—when they talked about it, which wasn't often—were syphilis and gonorrhea. Those two diseases are still alive and well. But today's doctors have identified over twenty genital infections that are known to be spread through sexual contact.

Venereal Diseases

Sexually transmitted diseases are rampaging all around us.[5] One authority has said that only the common cold is spreading faster than gonorrhea. Three million cases of sexually transmitted diseases are reported to health authorities in the United States each year. And it's getting worse. One million Americans contract gonorrhea each year. Twenty-one million suffer from genital herpes. And AIDS has burst upon the world like an ancient Egyptian plague, threatening to destroy millions of lives in the coming decades.

One hundred thousand cases of syphilis are reported annually. In one large Midwestern metropolitan area, the cases of syphilis more than doubled between 1989 and 1990.[6] There were five times as many cases in 1990 as there had been in 1988. The largest increase of syphilis in that city was not among homosexuals, but among heterosexuals.

Most people do not realize that they have VD until sometime after it has invaded their bodies. The reason for that is that many of these diseases—certainly the most common, gonorrhea and syphilis—often are not immediately accompanied by telltale symptoms. If left untreated, both of these diseases can cause insanity and death.

Gonorrhea and syphilis can be cured by penicillin-type drugs. Herpes Simplex II can be treated for relief of symptoms, but, as yet, it cannot be cured. Herpes will not kill a person, but it will make one painfully ill from time to time. A cure for AIDS has not been discovered either; AIDS is always fatal.

STDs that have been contracted by sexual intercourse are often passed on to the children of women who are infected. In major cities in our country hospitals are trying to care for hundreds of babies who are born with AIDS. Tiny babies also can get syphilis from their mothers. In fact, the disease is transmitted to preborn children in 70-100% of the cases where the mother is infected. Often this causes the baby to be born dead or with severe birth defects.

The Best Way to Stay Healthy

But you can be *absolutely sure* that venereal disease will never strike you, except, perhaps, under extremely rare circumstances. How? Remain a virgin until you marry, marry a virgin, and enjoy a relationship in which you are sexually faithful to each other.

Almost 100% of the people who have STDs today caught those diseases by having sex with someone who was infected. Some people with AIDS are exceptions. AIDS can be caught from infected hypodermic needles. In rare cases, medical laboratory technicians and recipients of blood transfusions have been infected by AIDS after coming into contact with contaminated blood. But such cases account for only a very small portion (less than 1%) of all those with AIDS. None of these diseases can be caught from toilet seats, drinking glasses, or mosquitoes. These diseases are spread by sexual contact.

If you obey God's design for sex and associate with people who do the same, you do not need to fear these diseases.

Protecting Yourself

Many believe it is foolish to encourage people to quit having sexual intercourse with many different partners. There are people who believe that the best way to stop the spread of STDs is to educate people to use condoms during sex. That's why "protected sex" (sex using a condom) is stressed.

A condom is a latex covering (it looks like a long balloon) which is pulled over a penis before sexual intercourse. Condoms, some say, will prevent those sexually transmitted diseases from being passed on. Unfortunately, condoms have a high failure rate both because they are used incorrectly and because they are manufactured poorly. At least one out of ten condoms fails.

An article in *Newsweek* (August 31, 1987, p. 72) warns against trusting condoms too much for protection from disease. It quotes Dr. Helen Singer Kaplan, director of the Human Sexuality Program at New York Hospital. She said, "Although lab studies have demonstrated that latex condoms block the entry of the AIDS virus, there is no scientific proof that they do so during intercourse. Furthermore . . . the protection they provide against AIDS could be considerably lower, since the virus is many times smaller than the human sperm. Also, a woman can get pregnant only a few days each month but is at risk for AIDS every time she has sex with an infected partner."

Protected Sex Is Not God's Way

God warned us against sexual activity outside of marriage. One of the reasons for that warning was to keep us from being exposed to venereal disease. God does not allow for sexual activity outside of marriage as long as you "protect" yourself. Even people who don't care about God's will should know that that doesn't work—for any length of time anyway. Just look at what's happening. Even with all the talk about "protected sex," VD continues to spread.

Isn't it unfortunate that many educated people don't recognize that God was deadly serious when he told us that sexual intercourse is only for married people to enjoy with each other? Isn't it sad that people continue to try to find ways to get around God's design for sexual intercourse? In the end those folks just bring harm to themselves and others.

But even if we could be sexually active and be assured that we wouldn't "get caught" by catching some disease or causing a pregnancy, we who know Jesus as our Savior would still want to use sex as God designed it to be used. Living according to God's plan for us is the way we express our gratitude for his forgiveness and love. The Bible encourages us, "Be imitators of God, therefore, as dearly loved children, and live a life of love, just as Christ loved us and gave himself for us as a fragrant offering and sacrifice to God" (Ephesians 5:1,2).

Precious Father, you had many reasons for restricting sexual intercourse to married couples. I pray for the millions of people who did not pay attention to your will and now are paying the price, some with their lives. Use their sickness to draw them closer to you. And help me to want to honor your instructions about my sexuality and to encourage others to do the same, not only because of the harm that breaking your laws causes, but because you have loved me so much in your Son.

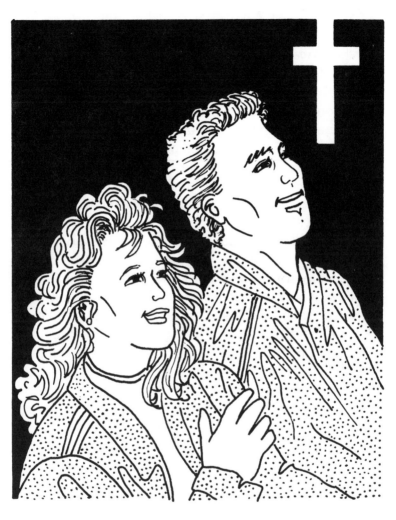

10.

HERE IT COMES

When I was in seventh grade, there was a girl I liked a lot. I don't remember anymore exactly what it was that I liked about Suzy, but I do remember that she was about six inches taller than I was.

Early adolescence is a crazy time. We go through a host of changes. Our bodies grow. We begin feeling emotions and sensations we never felt before. The opposite sex seems more and more important. We feel more and more like adults, but at times we'd just as soon be kids again.

We and all our friends are changing. But nobody is changing at the same rate as anybody else. Some people blossom into adult-looking bodies while all their classmates still look like kids. Some people still have kid-looking bodies while all their classmates look like adults. Some girls think guys are the greatest thing to happen to them since they discovered candy. Other girls couldn't care less about guys. The same extremes are true of guys.

So what kinds of changes can you expect during your teen years? This chapter talks about the physical changes you can anticipate. The next chapter helps you understand the changes you'll need to grow through on the way to emotional maturity.

Girl Changes

Girls are about six months ahead of boys as they develop the ability to reproduce. However, girls usually begin to grow into their adult bodies about two years before boys start growing into theirs. Girls' growth spurts happen between age ten and a half and fourteen. Because growth often takes place in spurts (short bursts of rapid growth), teenage girls can require more sleep than when they were younger.

Breast development begins three or four years before their first period (menarche). Pubic hair appears one and a half to two and a half years before menarche. And underarm hair appears about six months before the first period.

Skin tends to be oilier during this time, and that can cause pimples (acne). The amount of acne you will have is determined in large measure by the genes your parents passed on to you. You can minimize it, however, by keeping your face extra clean.

Girls entering puberty will also notice that they perspire more. Their sweat glands are beginning to work on an adult level. Deodorants will cover the smell (take the odor away). Antiperspirants will stop the wetness. Each person must determine whether deodorants or antiperspirants work best for her.

A girl's body may begin to produce eggs (ovulate) before her first period, but ovulation and menstruation usually happen together about three quarters of the way through her growth spurt. Girls have reached puberty when menarche occurs. Be sure to read Chapter Eight on menstruation entitled "Monthly Preparations for New Life."

All these changes are brought on when the body's endocrine system of glands kicks in. At some point the hypothalamus in the brain sends a signal to the pituitary gland, the key gland in the endocrine system, that it's time to turn this child's body into an adult body. The production of estrogen and progesterone begins in the ovaries as they ripen into almond sized organs. Those hormones act on the body to broaden hips, develop breasts, cause the sexual organs to grow and mature, and initiate some size and weight gain.

Boy Changes

The endocrine system brings about the same kind of maturing in boys. Boys reach puberty when they are first able to ejaculate. That normally happens three to four months after coarse, curly hair replaces the downy hair in their pubic areas. The ability to ejaculate usually is achieved near the peak of their growth spurt. That spurt generally occurs between age twelve and a half and sixteen, with major growth taking place during age fourteen. About a year before ejaculation is possible, the penis and testicles begin to grow and ready themselves for their role in reproduction.

Some boys notice that their breasts enlarge. This is a common and temporary part of growing into adulthood. When puberty has been reached, hair begins to grow thicker and darker on the arms and legs, under the arms, and in the pubic area, including the scrotum. Facial hair begins to sprout. Some teenage boys need to begin to shave rather early. Other can put off shaving until their later teen years. Shaving regularly will not cause the hair to grow back darker or heavier. A person's genes determine that.

The male voice begins to deepen as puberty sets in. Some teenage boys find that they can't trust how their voice will sound when they speak or especially when they sing during this adjustment period. That, too, is part of growing into adulthood and is nothing to be embarrassed about.

Acne (facial pimples) is more of a problem for boys than for girls. Adolescent skin contains more oils. These oils tend to block skin pores and produce pimples. Acne can be reduced by washing, but it cannot be eliminated. As with girls, the amount of acne one has is greatly determined by his genes. Teens would probably find it interesting to ask their parents about the amount of acne they had.

Teenage boys will also discover that their sweat glands are more active than before. Regular showers and daily washing will be necessary to avoid body odor. The use of deodorants or antiperspirants is also important.

Wet Dreams

Wet dreams, also called nocturnal emissions, are a common experience for teenage boys. In the chapter entitled "The Male Half of the Reproductive System" we learned that the seminal vesicles are the storage place for sperm. God has provided wet dreams to release some of that sperm when the seminal vesicles are full.

During a wet dream the teenager usually finds himself in a sexually stimulating situation. Those thoughts are caused by the higher than normal hormone level created when the seminal vesicles are full. The penis becomes erect and an ejaculation takes place. The teenager will feel orgasm and a sense of relief because his hormone level has fallen.

Often boys are embarrassed by their wet dreams. These emissions are, however, entirely normal. They are as much a part of growing up as a deepening voice, facial hair, and broadening shoulders. This is the body's method for releasing built-up sperm and a part of being male.

But aren't sexually explicit dreams sinful? Yes, they are; just as lust-filled daydreaming is sinful. That's another reason we value Jesus so highly. His crucifixion forgives us—even for the misuse of sexuality that happens in our dreams.

Sexual Urges

When puberty sets in, teens become more and more aware of the opposite sex and their attraction to that gender. Not everyone will experience to the same degree the desire to develop a close relationship with a member of the opposite sex. That's OK. It is just as normal to be interested in the opposite sex as it is not to be interested.

For most teens, however, sexual thoughts will enter their minds very regularly—even every few minutes—especially for boys. Since sexual thoughts will be new experiences, it will take some time and effort to learn to control them.

Being a teen and living in a body which is now physically ready for sexual relations can seem like driving a street-legal dragster. You know your car could burst away from a stop light and leave all the other cars in its dust, but you also know that speeding is illegal. You need to wait to squeal away from a stop until you are on the dragway, where it is legal. When puberty begins, you are capable of having sex and producing children, but God has established guidelines for us to use that gift. We'll need to harness our sexual urges until our circumstances fit God's guidelines.

In the meantime, what should you do with those sexual thoughts that keep popping into your head? Here are several suggestions.

1. Thank God that you are normal. God has equipped us with a sex drive. There's nothing sinful about that. In fact, it's a wonderful gift of his love. Sin gets involved when we misuse that sex drive.

2. Whenever you have a lustful thought, don't grab it in your mind and play with it. Rather dismiss it by saying to yourself, "Thank you, Father, for allowing me to reject improper thoughts. I reject this thought in the name of Jesus Christ."

3. Each time you catch yourself mulling sexual thoughts in your mind,ask God for the forgiveness Jesus won for you on the cross and guarantees you in his resurrection. Remind yourself of David's experience with sin in Psalm 32:5, "I said, 'I will confess my transgressions to the Lord'—and you forgave the guilt of my sin." Claim God's promise in 1 John 1:9, "If we confess our sins, he is faithful and just and will forgive us our sins and purify us from all unrighteousness."

4. Rejoice over the smaller victories. If the only time you will allow yourself to feel good is when you have completely eliminated lust from your life, you won't ever smile again. Keep track of your minor wins over sexual thoughts and thank God for them.

5. Determine what things or situations stimulate sexu-

al thoughts in you. Perhaps a certain television program, magazine, or place (a swimming pool?) churns up lustful thoughts. Steer clear of as many of those situations as you can; guard your thoughts when you must be in those situations.

6. Arm yourself with God's word and prayer. Be sure to set aside time each day to read and think about God's word and to talk with your Father in prayer.

Father, you've said I should thank you in all circumstances. I thank you for the changes that are happening in my body. These changes make me feel strange and wonderful all at the same time. I feel confused sometimes and ready for anything at others. I'm kind of living on the edge. That's all right, because I know you are there to protect me and to catch me when I fall. I thank you for designing me to change like this—as you make me into an adult. But I especially thank you that you have loved mr enough to make me youd dear child by sending Jesus to be my Savior.

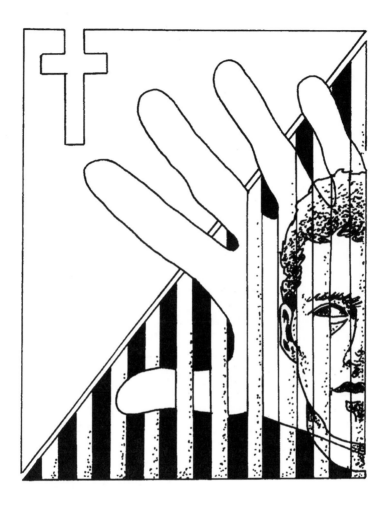

11.

SOLO SEX

If you do it you'll go blind. Or you might start growing long hair all over your body. Or you might age faster than normal. Or you could get epilepsy. Or you'll destroy brain cells; you'll lose your memory; you might even go insane.

Those are some of the scary things people used to believe would happen as a result of masturbation. But what's the truth about masturbation? How should we Christians feel about it? And, if it's wrong, what do we do to overcome it?

Those are the items we're going to tackle in this chapter.

What is Masturbation?

Masturbation is the touching, stroking, fondling of one's own genitals in order to produce a pleasant sexual sensation. It is also called autoeroticism and self sexual stimulation. Some have misunderstood the sin of Onan in Genesis 38:9,10 as a form of masturbation and have called masturbation "onanism."

Both males and females are able to masturbate. In fact studies have shown that almost all boys (98%) have masturbated by the time they reach college age. The percentage of girls is only slightly behind that (80%).

Adolescents usually practice masturbation to comfort themselves when they are feeling low, to feel better about themselves when the pressure is on, and to release pent-up sexual energy. Some teens use masturbation for a psychological rush in order to feel good about themselves in the same way as others use food. There are people who suggest that teens should masturbate as a way of discovering how their genitals work.

Medical studies have proven that masturbation will cause no physical harm. In fact, masturbation will not hurt a person's body even if it is done repeatedly.

There are, however, some emotional and scriptural concerns about masturbation which you need to know. Let's talk about the scriptural concerns first.

What Does God Say?

The Bible does not specifically mention masturbation. Nowhere in Scripture is masturbation listed by name as a sin. But that does not mean that it is pleasing to our Father, for the Scriptures do speak about lust—and lust goes hand in hand with masturbation. Lust is thinking sexual thoughts about someone who is not your husband or wife. The Scriptures tell us lust is sinful.

The Bible says that lust is something unbelievers do (Ephesians 4:17-19, 1 Peter 4:3). Unfortunately, Christians cannot completely overcome sinful lust either. God tells us that lust comes from our sinful nature, the old adam, and is a form of idolatry (Colossians 3:5).

Jesus said, "Anyone who looks at a woman lustfully has already committed adultery with her in his heart" (Matthew 5:28). Paul tells us to avoid any kind of sexual immorality including lust: "It is God's will that you should be sanctified [that means, live a holy life]: that you should avoid sexual immorality; that each of you should learn to control his own body in a way that is holy and honorable, not in passionate lust like the heathen, who do not know God" (1 Thessalonians 4:3-5).

It's no wonder, then, that the Bible says lust is not part of God's plan to provide us with pleasure. Actually, it's a spiritual roadblock that the sin-filled world puts in our path. "For everything in the world—the cravings of sinful man, the lust of his eyes and the boasting of what he has and does—comes not from the Father but from the world" (1 John 2:16).

Allowing lust to occupy our minds robs us of time and energy—which we could use more productively to serve our Savior and his people. Lust puts God in second place in our lives.

Lust can easily sidetrack us from dealing with important issues in our lives. Sometimes people hide from reality by creating their own world inside their minds, where everything works just the way they want it. If we allow ourselves to think sexual thoughts all the time, we won't have any time to consider how to tackle our problems, face our fears, and plan for the future.

Lust also causes us to view people as things we want to use to satisfy our selfish feelings. The picture of a naked person in a pornographic magazine doesn't help us say, "Lord, thank you for creating such beauty in the human body" or "Here is a person Jesus died to save. I wonder how I can help her/him get closer to Jesus." Those pictures lead us to think about how we would like to use that person to make us feel good.

And that brings us to a final Scripture consideration about masturbation. God wants us to know who is in charge in our lives. "A man is a slave to whatever has mastered him," God says in 2 Peter 2:19. If sexual thoughts and masturbation are out of our control, we are their slaves and they our masters. Then Jesus is being pushed aside as our Lord.

More than that, if we are spending time dreaming up sexually stimulating situations, we're not doing that to his glory (1 Corinthians 10:31). That's why we're told, "Flee the evil desires of youth, and pursue righteousness, faith, love and peace, along with those who call on the Lord out of a pure heart" (2 Timothy 2:22).

A littler later in this chapter, we're going to talk about how to "flee the evil desires of youth," but before we do, you need to know how masturbation affects the way we teach ourselves to think about sex.

How Does It Shape Our View of Sex?

Outside of spiritual reasons for avoiding masturbation, are there other reasons not to masturbate?

Although, it is true that masturbation will cause no physical harm to a person, it may condition a male to come to orgasm too quickly. This may result in premature ejaculation during sexual intercourse. That means that a male reaches orgasm before he is able to insert his penis into his partner's vagina or that it occurs during insertion. A woman's sexual pleasure is greatly diminished when this happens.

Masturbation can also warp the way we look at the blessings of sex. Do you remember how we talked about the reasons God gave sexual intimacy to humans in the chapter called "Here's What It's All

About"? We learned that sex blesses us with freedom from loneliness, with pleasure, and with children. One of the problems with masturbation is that it does not free us from loneliness, because it is solo sex. It can teach us that sexual pleasure is something we should get out of sexual activity rather than something we should be giving to someone else. Masturbation can teach us to be sexually selfish.

Masturbation uses for one person a blessing God intended to be used by a married heterosexual (male/female) couple. People who masturbate excessively as teens can begin to feel that sex is best when experienced alone. These people may find it difficult to relate sexually to their spouse.

Masturbation can never really satisfy because it cannot bring an end to our loneliness. It takes a very powerful urge for an intimate relationship with someone of the opposite sex and turns it back on itself. That kind of sex only makes a person feel more isolated.

Guilt often accompanies masturbation. Although masturbation, like every sin, has been atoned for on the cross, sometimes Christians have a hard time accepting their forgiveness. That guilt may cause a person to feel unworthy, even worthless. It can cause a person to believe that there is something wrong about sexual intercourse even within marriage.

Since sexual thoughts and masturbation are fueled by pornography, excessive masturbation may teach a person that he can become sexually aroused only by pornographic magazines or films. This will certainly hinder a sexual relationship with one's spouse.

How to Conquer It

If you have never masturbated, don't start. A person who has never masturbated is just as normal sexually as those who have.

Many Christian young people struggle with masturbation, however. They may find that it can bring excitement and pleasure, but they may also learn that it can also bring guilt and a yearning for deliverance.

Teens need to know that they don't have to masturbate. They can stop. Nothing bad will happen to them. Their bodies might be saying, "You have to! You have to or you'll explode or something." But bodies that tell people that are lying. Folks who masturbate are not helpless victims; they can conquer their habit.

Here are some things to share with someone who is struggling with overcoming masturbation:

1. Stop hating yourself. The lust that goes along with masturbation is a sin, but it is no worse than any other sin. It does not make you a more terrible person than anger, greed, or hate does. God stands ready to welcome you into his open, loving arms. It's good that you feel sorry for what you've done, but you also need to know that God forgives you for Jesus' sake.

2. Confess your sin to God and ask him to forgive you because Jesus is your Savior. "If we confess our sins, he is faithful and just and will forgive us our sins and purify us from all unrighteousness" 1 John 1:9). Do this each time you give in to lust.

3. Thank God that he has given you sexual feelings.

They are a gift which will allow you to experience great blessing after you are married. Praise God because you trust that a day is coming when he will empower you to harness the sex drive he has given you.

4. Don't just commit yourself to *try* to stop. Commit yourself to stop. "Try" is a weasel word. It says, "My heart really isn't in this. I'm probably not going to do it. But I'll make an effort." It is better to make up your mind that with God's help and blessing you *will* conquer masturbation. If/when you fail, you simply start over again.

5. Avoid the things that encourage you to masturbate. By the time you have begun an act of masturbation, it can be extremely hard to stop. So rather than determining not to masturbate, think about what leads you to the act: pornographic videos and magazines, spending time alone in your room, etc. Avoid those things by doing something else (go out with your friends, take up a new sport, go to a Bible study).

6. Recognize that God has the power to deliver you from masturbation. If he has chosen not to do that right now, it may be because there is another area of your life he wants to deal with first, such as your temper, your lack of responsibility, your failure to worship. That doesn't mean you should give up the struggle, but it may mean you need to struggle harder in another area of your life. Search out God's plan for you.

Hang in There

A young friend asked me why God builds teens with sexual desires. "Wouldn't it have been better if we didn't get those feelings until after we were married?" she asked. It might seem that would be better, but God had another plan. We need our teen years to learn how to control our drive for sexual fulfillment.

Regulating our sexual urges is like learning to play a musical instrument. A lot of time and hard work go into being able to play an acceptable solo before an auditorium filled with people. During our teen years—and for many also during their early twenties—we are given time to learn how to control our sex drive so we're ready to use it when married.

There will be pressures on you during your teen years to try masturbation. Your friends may tease you if you admit you haven't "done it" yet. You'll probably also feel your hormones urging you on to "give it a shot." I hope you won't give in.

But if you do, don't become discouraged. When you fail in your struggle, repeat the steps that I've just listed and start over again. Just don't give up as you fight with this problem.

Father, I thank you for creating me with sexual urges. I know that you have many wonderful blessings to give me because I am a sexual creature. But for now, Lord, I need your help in standing up against the pressures of my peers on the outside and my hormones on the inside to give in to lustful thoughts and actions. By your Spir-

it's power be a mighty fortress around me so that none of Satan's demons can move me to lust. Help me to control my sex drive so that I keep you first in my life and praise you for loving and saving me.

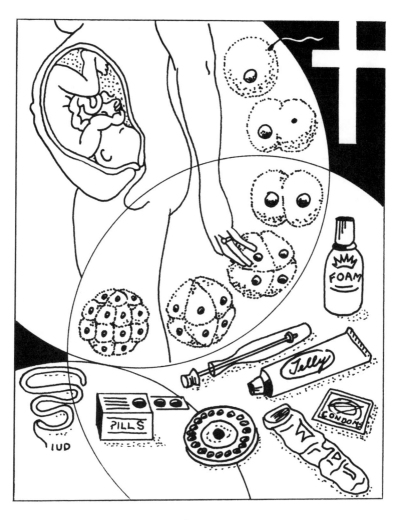

12.

PREGNANCY AND CONTRACEPTION

I admit it. Back in junior high school when I was struggling to get all the facts straight about how life begins, I thought that every time a man and woman had sex they would have a child.

Of course, that isn't true. Conception is possible for a woman for only a few hours each month. Even when couples have sex during that time, there is no guarantee that a new life will be conceived. In the end, it is God who decides when to grant life to another human being, not we.

You should know, however, that pregnancy can occur the first time a woman has sexual relations. It may also happen at any time during her monthly cycle, not just in the middle of it. And it certainly can happen without the woman experiencing orgasm.

Contraception

There are methods available for preventing the conception of children. These are properly called contraceptives (contra means "against"; -ceptive is an abbreviation for "conception"). There are also birth control methods that work after a baby has been conceived by killing the tiny girl or boy. These are called abortifacients.

Methods that prevent conception include

- **condoms**, a latex covering that fits over the penis and stops the sperm from entering the vagina. A slang word for condom is rubber.

- **spermicides**, which are sprayed into the vagina before sexual intercourse so they kill the sperm that are deposited there.

104

- **diaphragms and contraceptive sponges**, which are inserted into the vagina before intercourse to block the passage of sperm into the cervix.

- **natural family planning**, which calculates the most likely time during the month for an egg to be present in the wife. During that time, couples do not have sex.

- **sterilization**. In men this is called vasectomy; in women it is called a tubal ligation or having one's tubes tied. Although doctors have had limited success with reversing these operations, people who think about getting a vasectomy or tubal ligation need to consider that that operation will make them permanently incapable of having children.

With the exception of a properly done sterilization, none of these methods is 100% effective. Most of them are somewhat ineffective. The diaphragm is reported to be up to 97% effective. However, that is under ideal conditions. In normal use it has been found to be as low as 70% effective. That means it offers no protection from pregnancy about one out of three times a couple has sex. Condoms, in normal use, are effective in as little as 80% of the time; they offer no protection from pregnancy about one out of five times.[7] For people who are sexually promiscuous, condoms have been recommended because they help to stop the spread of venereal disease. There is evidence, however, that condoms do not offer as much protection as is necessary. See chapter nine, "It Can Make You Sick."

Another method of contraception which has a high degree of failure is withdrawal of the penis from the vagina before the male reaches orgasm. There are three reasons this method does not work well. First, it is hard to time the orgasm so the penis is withdrawn before ejaculation into the vagina. Second, some sperm are usually released by the penis a few minutes before orgasm takes place. Finally, there is a lack of emotional and sexual satisfaction for both partners.

Abortifacients

Methods which end up destroying the life of a newly conceived child are called abortifacients since they cause very early abortions. These methods include

- **IUDs or Intra-Uterine Devices**. These devices are made of a coil of twisted wire. Doctors insert an IUD into the uterus. There a woman's normal movements cause the IUD to irritate the walls of the womb. Because of that mild inflammation of the womb, a new life will not be able to implant itself on the side of the uterus, and it will die.

- **The Pill**. Birth control pills are designed to work in three ways. First, they prevent eggs from ripening (ovulation). They also cause chemical changes in the mucus of the cervix so sperm cannot pass into the uterus. In some cases, however, conception still happens. The Pill works in another way to deal with that. It makes the walls of the uterus hard so that a newly conceived child will not be able to implant itself there. That tiny child will then die and be flushed out of the mother's body. Birth control pills are available only through doctors. No one should ever take someone else's birth control pills. These pills must also be taken for a number of weeks before they become effective.

- **Norplant**. This form of birth control is designed to work in a woman's body in the same way as the Pill. Matchstick-sized silicone capsules are implanted beneath the skin of a woman's upper arm. Over the course of five years they slowly release birth-controlling hormones.

- **The Morning After Pill**. In some parts of the world a pill is now available which a woman takes after having sex. The chemicals in the pill kill any fertilized eggs contained in the woman's Fallopian tubes.

- **Abortion**. Almost all abortions in our country are done on women whose pre-born children are eight to ten weeks from conception. We noted in Chapter Five, "Once Upon A Time," how obviously human those lives are.

None of these methods of stopping pregnancy should be used by Christian husbands and wives, because they result in the murder of the youngest of children. Since life begins at conception, God's Fifth Commandment obligates us to protect life from that point.

Sometimes Christians use one of these methods for contraception without realizing how it works. Those believers will find great comfort in God's promise, "There is now no condemnation for those who are in Christ Jesus" (Romans 8:1). God's forgiveness will also motivate them to find an acceptable form of contraception.

You should also know that the Pill and the IUD are not 100% effective in stopping pregnancy. The Pill has an 11% failure rate. That means if 100 teenage girls are on the Pill and are sexually active, 11 will become pregnant this year. The IUD has a failure rate of almost 11%.[8] (And here's something else about the Pill. Researchers have found that young women who take the Pill increase their risk of developing breast cancer.)[9]

Homemade Methods

Some teens believe they can make their own contraceptives. This is not true. A plastic bag or plastic wrap is no substitute for a condom. A woman's jumping up and down after intercourse will not prevent pregnancy. Neither will douching with cola or any other liquid following sexual relations. If anything, such douching encourages infection. Drinking ice cold water will not kill the sperm which have entered a woman's body either.Don't allow anyone to convince you that contraception can be accomplished in any way other than those ways mentioned above. Many women who believed those myths are now mothers.

Why Married Couples Use Contraceptives

There are four principles married couples will want to consider about using contraceptives. The first is that children are a blessing God gives. The second is that God, not humans, determines when children will be conceived. The third is that we are to be good stewards of everything God has given us. The fourth is that everything we do should show our trust in God. Let's talk about that.

Right after God created Adam and Eve, he blessed them by giving them the privilege of producing children. He told them to "be fruitful and increase in number" (Genesis 1:28). The Bible always talks about children as God's special blessing to married couples. Psalm 127 says, "Sons are a heritage from the LORD, children a reward from him. Like arrows in the hands of a warrior are sons born in one's youth. Blessed is the man whose quiver is full of them." When Christian couples think about using contraceptives, they must carefully consider how God wants to bless them with children. Will the use of contraceptives frustrate God's plan to increase their happiness with a family?

The second principle married couples will consider is that they really don't control when their children will be conceived. As much as some people might think they can *plan* their families, it is God who decides when to create a new human being, not we. The psalmist says about God, "You created my inmost being; you knit me together in my mother's womb. I praise you because I am fearfully and wonderfully made; your works are wonderful, I know that full well" Psalm 139:13,14. The prophet Jeremiah testifies, "The word of the Lord came to me, saying,...'I formed you in the womb' (Jeremiah 1:4,5). Married couples who are Christians will recognize that they don't produce children by having sex. God creates life when he pleases.

Christians want to make the best use of everything God has given them to thank God for his love. They will use their intelligence, their money, their abilities, their home, their bodies—everything—to bring God honor. That's being a good steward. Sometimes being a good steward means not doing things, like not eating too much. Food is certainly a blessing God has given us, but too much food ruins our bodies. Children, too, are a blessing, but sometimes it may be better to avoid having children. For example, sometimes a pregnancy threatens the life of a mother; sometimes a mother or father cannot emotionally handle another child; sometimes parents cannot afford to provide for additional children.

But whenever Christian parents think they are in a situation that calls for attempting to restrict the size of their family, they must carefully weigh how much their decision is based on a lack of trust in God. That's the fourth principle. Sometimes parents decide to have only one or two children so they "can give them the best." But that may mean those parents selfishly want material things for themselves and they are unwilling to share with more than a child or two. That's a lack of trust in God, who has told us that every child is a blessing, not a burden. That's not fully trusting the God who has adopted us into his family by sacrificing his Son for us.

To use or not to use contraceptives is a major decision. Married couples who love their Lord should not hastily arrive at such a decision. They need to pray over the matter. They should seek advice from other sincere Christians. They need to evaluate their motives for wanting to limit family size and determine whether they are God-pleasing. If Christian couples discover that their reasons for using contraceptives have been wrong, they need to claim God's forgiveness and to say thanks to God for his love by steering clear of that sin in the future.

A Reminder

This chapter on ways to stop pregnancy from happening, is not to help you be sexually active without "getting caught." It is to give you the information you need to make the right choices, the choices God wants you to make. If you didn't know about contraceptives and abortifacients, you would be more likely to misuse them. I also want you to help your friends with those choices. Without the proper information, they may easily be misled.

We Christians understand that contraceptives are for use by married couples who have prayerfully sought God's guidance about the size and timing of their families. Contraceptives should never have to be used by unmarried people, because unmarried people should not be sexually active. That's what God wants—and that's what we who have been forgiven by him want too.

Father, Creator of life, I realize that it is good for me to know the difference between contraception and birth control. I also need to be aware of the things married couples should consider about using contraceptives. Use me to help my friends

understand these things, especially to understand how contraceptive devices need never be used by young people who are doing your will, because young people who are doing your will are not sexually active.

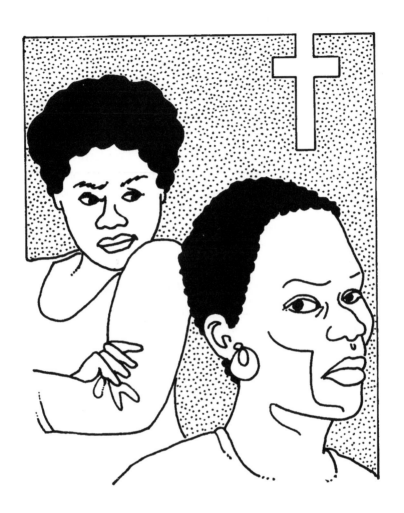

13.

More Than Growing; Maturing

"No. I don't want to go. I've got plans."

The subject was the family vacation. My object was to avoid it. Somehow, spending two weeks camping with my parents, two brothers, and a sister was not my idea of fun. I'd be away from my friends and cooped up with my family. I was "too mature," I thought, to enjoy another dumb family vacation.

I ended up going. I also made myself miserable—and my family along with me—for the first day or two. It seemed the mature thing to do at the time. But it doesn't anymore.

Emotional Maturity

There comes a point when our bodies are finished developing. After that we won't get any taller, our voice won't get any deeper, our reproductive organs won't get more productive. But there never comes a point when we have fully developed emotionally. Maturing is a lifelong process. Nonetheless, it's a process that needs a good start during our teen years.

Growing into adulthood is much more than getting to live in an adult body. A maturing adult is someone who —

- **recognizes the kind of person it is that God intended him/her to be**. God has made us all unique. He has made us his children through his Son. But more than that. He has made each of us for a special purpose that no one else could accomplish as well as we can. Every Christian is the right tool for a job God wants done.

  A maturing person has investigated his talents and abilities and knows what special gifts of the

Spirit God has granted him (Romans 12:3-8; 1 Corinthians 12:7-11).

- **is content with being the person God has made him**. God hasn't made everyone to be rich, beautiful, and famous. But everyone of us is important. The maturing person is happy to serve in God's world according to God's design for him because he knows how much his Father loves him (Ephesians 2:10; Hebrews 13:5).

- **is striving to develop all the potential that God has given him**. When a person knows why God put him on this planet and is content with that, he'll want to be the best at whatever God has designed him to be. That striving for excellence is the believer's way of thanking God for his love and forgiveness (1 Corinthians 10:31; Philippians 3:7-11).

That's what a mature individual is like. To arrive at that point, however, will require some work. Unfortunately, some people aren't willing to join in that struggle. I know a man in his mid-thirties who hasn't grown beyond early teen levels of maturity. Even though he is married and has children, he changes jobs every few months, smokes pot, and can't live on his budget. If he feels like taking a day off from work, he calls in sick without giving much thought to how his family will manage on less income or how his creditors will feel about not getting paid.

Maturing means being responsible for yourself and those you have committed yourself to. Many times a maturing person will carry out a job he dislikes simply because he said he'd do it or because others are depending on him to get it done. Think about what that means when—

- you tell your parents you'll be available on a Friday night for some family time only to find that you've been invited to a party that night.

- you are elected to student council at school but your friends think all the people on the student council are dorks.

- you agree to go shopping with one friend, but another friend asks you to go to a movie with her.

The "Tween" Years

The teen years have been called the "tween" years, the years between childhood and adulthood. During this part of your life you'll have times when you'll want to be treated like an adult. At other times you'll prefer escaping that responsibility and being treated like a child. That's permissible—although the older you get, the more you should be willing to carry the responsibility that goes with being an adult.

Because the teen years are a "tween" time, it is not unusual for teenagers to feel confused about themselves, their goals in life, and their reason for living. In a way, the cards are stacked against teens feeling good about themselves just because of the changes they are going through.

Oily skin produces blackheads and acne. Growth spurts make a person uncoordinated for a while and quite self-conscious. Shower rooms at school force a teen to compare himself with his peers and often make him depressed because there are others who are more developed than he is. Cruel comments by classmates add to poor self-esteem.

A teenage body surges with changing levels of hormones. These body-built chemicals warp the way adolescents view life. There are days when tears come easily and times when bullheadedness takes over. The new emotions teens feel take a while to adjust to. Sometimes they catch teens off-guard and cause problems. Learn from your ups and downs. But don't think you're going crazy. You're just growing up.

The confusion and frustration may seem even worse because building relationships is important to teens. This process helps teens grow into adults who can work well with others and who will choose wisely when finding a lifelong mate. But a number of things get in the way of relationships during adolescence. For example,

- Everyone matures at a different rate, so a teen might feel "out of it" when he's with his school friends because they are not as far along or are further along than he is.

- Relationships are tested and sometimes destroyed because of immaturity. Teens are not always ready to keep up their end of the bargain in a relationship.

- Looking good becomes a high priority to teens; a hair out of place, a spot on a blouse, or a pimple may destroy a teen's sense of self-esteem. Most teens wish they could change their looks in some way: a different nose, broader shoulders, becoming taller/shorter, etc.

- Some teens become very shy for fear of saying something embarrassing which might ruin a relationship. Others try to cover their fear of embarrassment by talking continuously.

Being a teenager can have some rocky moments. But that's all normal. It's all part of growing up. It's something everyone goes through.

The teen years are an excellent time for a person to discover that good feelings about oneself can't be based on what one looks like, on the crowd of people one associates with, or on one's abilities (athletic, academic, or others). The only thing that will enable us to feel good about who we are is recognizing whom God has made us.

Discovery Time

The teen years are a time for discovering who it is that God has made you, for finding your niche in life, for exploring roles to find which ones fit you and which ones don't. It's not only OK to experiment with different kinds of clothes, hairstyles, subjects in school, and sports during adolescence; it's important that you do that.

We discover what kind of tool the Lord has built us to be as we find out what we like to do and what we're good at (those two things aren't always the same). We also get some ideas about how God wants to use us as others give us some feedback on the things we're doing. The things people compliment us on are probably areas God wants us to pursue. But we'll never really know what we like to do, what we're good at, or what people will compliment us for unless we try a variety of things.

By the way, it's perfectly OK to try something and fail. That's part of God's way of helping you define who you are—or who you aren't.

But beware. There will always be a temptation to want to explore the unhealthy areas of life as well as the healthy. Many have tried to explore the dangerous world of alcohol, drugs, smoking, sex, and partying— thinking they could do it without harm. Few come away without having been hurt. A tragic number are destroyed.

How can you know what to explore and what to steer clear of? Jesus tells us he has given us the Holy Spirit to counsel us ("The Counselor, the Holy Spirit, whom the Father will send in my name, will teach you all things and will remind you of everything I have said to you" (John 14:26). Keep your relationship with the Spirit strong by staying in touch with his word during your teen years. Let God help you decide which areas you can investigate and which you need to avoid.

Conflict with Parents

The teen years can bring with them some conflict between parents and teens. The reason: the teen years are a time of change. No change happens without some conflict. Change always requires giving up something you know for something you don't know.

During those "tween" years, teenagers, like a ping pong ball, bounce back and forth between wanting to enjoy childhood's lack of responsibility and wanting the benefits of adulthood. Teens often find it hard to figure out what side of the net to be on. Their hormone levels can vary greatly from day to day (hormones affect emotions). Body changes, emotional changes, and social changes team up to make teens feel quite insecure about themselves. It's no wonder that their parents can often be frustrated by that along with them.

You should also expect that some conflict will happen between you and your parents because of the change your parents are going through. That's right; your parents are struggling with change, too! It's a chore for most parents to adjust to the new adult relationships which are forming between them and their adolescent children. After thirteen years of being the authority figure to their children, parents find it hard to switch gears and make that slow transition from parent to friend as their children reach early adulthood.

That adjustment is complicated by the necessity teens often feel for choosing between their peers and their parents. And it gets more complicated. There will be times when you feel you need to choose between making your own decisions and living under the safety of your parents' wing. At other times you'll be torn between conforming to the standards of those around you and living up to your own values, which you want to be the same as God's values.

So expect that there will be times when you and your parents don't see eye to eye. But also remember that obedience to those in authority, even when those authority figures aren't acting in one's best interest, is a way of confessing our gratitude for Jesus. You've probably learned the Scripture passages that say,

"Children, obey your parents in the Lord, for this is right" (Ephesians 6:1) and "Children, obey your parents in everything, for this pleases the Lord" (Colossians 3:20).

Communicating with Parents

God-honoring obedience to parents does not mean you can't express your wishes to them. However, especially when emotions are running high, communication can be very tricky. Here are several ideas to help you improve your communication with your parents. You may want to show these ideas to your parents. That way they'll know the approach you'd like to take in talking with them.

1. When something about your parents is bothering you, don't do anything before you pray about it. Ask God to help you see the situation as he sees it.

2. Ask to speak with your parents. Make an appointment. Mutually agree on the place and time you will meet. You might say, "Mom and Dad, something has been bothering me about the way we've been getting along. Could we set a time to talk about it?"

3. Before your meeting, write down what you believe the problem is. Watch out for words like "always" and "never" (for example, "You never let me do anything with my friends"). Those words will get you talking about whether "always" or "never" is accurate rather than, for example, about your desire to spend more time with your friends. Also put yourself in your parents' shoes and write down

how you think they might see the situation. Remember to "speak the truth in love" (Ephesians 4:15), and "do not let any unwholesome talk come out of your mouths, but only what is helpful for building others up according to their needs, that it may benefit those who listen" (Ephesians 4:29). Note how you may have added to the problem.

4. When your meeting time arrives, calmly share with your parents what you have written. Listen as they react to your thoughts. To be sure you understand them, when they have finished reacting say, "I hear you saying that (for example) you don't want me to go out on Friday nights because I need to study more." Once you know you are understanding your parents' point, then you can share with them whether you agree or not.

5. Brainstorm ways that both the things you would like to happen and the things your parents want to happen might take place. When people brainstorm, they suggest as many ideas as possible without evaluating them. Every idea is written down, no matter how weird. When there are no more ideas, the list is evaluated for the most workable solutions. Often several ideas can be combined into one great idea.

6. Agree on one solution. You may even want to write down the role each person will have in making that solution a success.

7. Set another meeting time when you will evaluate how well the solution is working and make adjustments, if necessary.

8. Say thanks to your parents as they live up to their part of the solution. Don't forget to let them know how much you appreciate the way they are sticking to your agreement.

9 Don't wait for an issue to arise to talk with your parents. From time to time ask your parents about:

- their first date, dance, kiss, steady relationship
- what they felt best/worst about in high school
- when they felt most/least accepted in high school
- what they thought about living at home when they were growing up
- what they thought it would be like to be an adult
- what they wanted to do with their lives after high school
- what their parents thought about their friends
- who their idols were and why
- who their favorite teacher was
- who their favorite musicians were and the songs they liked the best.

Spiritual Maturity

It's interesting that the Bible connects emotional maturity and spiritual maturity. God tells us that we can't be emotionally mature unless we are spiritually mature. In fact, he says that the primary goal we Christians are striving for is to be mature and to help each other reach maturity.

Do you remember how it says in Ephesians 4:12,13 that God wants us Christians to be prepared to do "works of service, so that the body of Christ may be built up until we all reach unity in the faith and in the knowledge of the Son of God and become mature, attaining to the whole measure of the fullness of Christ"?

Did you notice how we become mature? When we are united in the true faith and when we really know Jesus. That means maturity happens only when we know God's word.

It's no wonder that the book of Hebrews scolds those Christians for not maturing by being in God's word and trusting it. "It is hard to explain [anything to you] because you are slow to learn. In fact, though by this time you ought to be teachers, you need someone to teach you the elementary truths of God's word all over again. You need milk, not solid food! Anyone who lives on milk, being still an infant, is not acquainted with the teaching about righteousness." Now listen as he goes on. "But solid food is for the mature, who by constant use have trained themselves to distinguish good from evil" (Hebrews 5:11-14).

Isn't that what it means to be mature? To be able to distinguish what is good from what is bad and to choose the good and reject the bad? God gives us that wisdom in his word. "If any of you lacks wisdom, he should ask God, who gives generously to all without finding fault, and it will be given to him" (James 1:5).

If you are really serious about becoming more mature, you need to listen to God.

It Has Nothing to Do with Size

The fact that a guy is six feet, six inches tall does not mean that he is grown up. The fact that a girl looks like she's twenty doesn't mean that she is mature. Emotional maturity is much different from physical maturity. It's also much more important.

Emotional maturity is a lifelong process. It's also a process we can't experience without developing spiritually. We need to work on emotional and spiritual maturing every day. It's always a challenge. But its rewards are worth it.

Heavenly Father, I want to be mature. But sometimes it seems too hard. My friends bug me. My parents get on my nerves. I frustrate myself. Help me to grow up—to grow up, not just on the outside, but on the inside. Help me get a handle on my emotions. I know I will do that only as I get to know you better. Keep me in your word. Keep me learning about you and your love, power, and wisdom. Keep me growing in my trust in you. Help me be more and more mature each day I live.

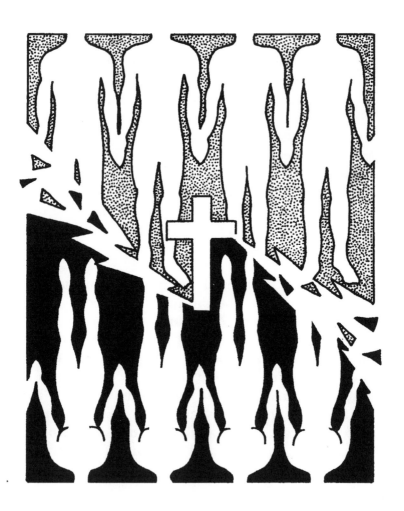

14.

SAME-SEX SEX

"Pastor, I've got something I need to tell you." With that Roger sat down in my office and slowly described a secret he had kept from everyone but his immediate family.

"I'm a homosexual. I have had sex with many men, starting back when I was in junior high. I dress up in women's clothing. And, I think, I'm rather attractive. Then I spend time on the streets of a neighboring city trying to be picked up by men. I've been arrested several times because cross-dressing is against the law here."

Roger looked like a pretty ordinary young man. He stood about five feet eight inches tall. He was slender and wore his hair fluffed out, almost like an afro. As he told me about his hidden life, I realized that there were some womanly traits he had which now made more sense. But I also realized that his traits were not out of the ordinary for a male. A number of "straight" men I knew acted more womanly than Roger.

He told me about some of the situations in which he had found himself. He had been beaten by his lovers and his lovers' friends. While lying to keep his secret identity under wraps, he had learned to lie about other things as well. He often used his lying ability to steal from his friends and family and to take advantage of his lovers. The story he told was filled with pain, rejection, fear, and abuse (physical, chemical, and sexual).

In this chapter we're going to talk about people like Roger who enjoy—sometimes are driven—by the desire to have sex with people of their own gender. We'll talk about why it's a sin and how we forgiven people are to relate to homosexuals.

A Definition

A homosexual act is an activity carried on between members of the same sex in order to produce orgasm. A homosexual is a man or woman who engages in homosexual acts. A homosexual woman is often called a lesbian. Studies have indicated that in the United States homosexual feelings may be present in as many as one out of ten individuals.

It is usually hard to recognize a homosexual. Although some homosexuals openly flaunt their sexual preference, most do not. It is a mistake—not to mention a sin against the Eighth Commandment—to think that a male who shows some feminine traits or a female who shows some masculine traits is homosexual. A man who enjoys sewing, cooking, and little babies is not necessarily a homosexual. A woman who is an avid hunter, baseball player, and mechanic is not necessarily a homosexual. Some homosexual men are heavily into "the manly arts" like competitive sports, body building, and car racing. Some homosexual women have children and seem to be great mothers, sew their own clothes, and don't have a single bulging muscle on their bodies.

Sexual intercourse between homosexuals is accomplished by stroking, petting, licking and sucking on the genitals of one's lover. A male homosexual will sometimes insert his penis into his partner's anus to reach orgasm.

Homosexuals have been calling themselves "gay" for a number of years. They feel it is a word which gives a more positive image to their lifestyle. Unfortunately, even a word like "gay" cannot hide the fact that homosexuality for most gays is not a happy experience. Homosexuals are not accepted or understood in our society, so they face much discrimination. They tend to suffer more than the average person from loneliness and rejection. Like Roger, they learn to lie, but those lies cause others not to trust them. Their homosexual friends often take advantage of them and tend not to be faithful to their promises. Worse, as a homosexual ages and he/she is not as physically attractive, the chances of finding a supportive partner decrease dramatically. And, of course, the ever-present fear of contracting AIDS and other STDs makes life for the homosexual one of continual insecurity.

Other Forms of Same-Sex Sex

Same-sex sex also takes other forms. Some individuals seems to enjoy heterosexual (male and female) sex as well as homosexual sex. These people are called bisexuals.

A transsexual is a person who feels trapped in a body of the wrong sex, a male in a female body or a female in a male body. They view their attraction to others of their sex not so much as homosexuality but as a natural attraction. They feel that deep within themselves they are the opposite sex of their body. For that reason, they tend not to be interested in relationships with homosexuals. Rather, they desire a relationship with a "straight" person. Some transsexuals have sex-change operations. That is an operation with a high failure rate and a hefty price tag.

A transvestite gets a sexual high from dressing up in clothing of the opposite sex. Most transvestites are married men who are not homosexual. In fact, most married transvestites have a good sexual relationship with their wives. They may continually wear an article of female clothing, like a bra or panties, under their regular clothes. Many of these men had unfortunate childhood experiences which led them to feel stimulated by cross-dressing.

The Reason People Are Homosexual

Psychiatrists do not agree about why people become homosexuals. It doesn't have anything to do with our bodies producing the wrong kind of hormones. Dr. John White, associate professor of psychiatry at the University of Manitoba and a well-know Christian author, says, "Our sex hormones do not necessarily determine either the kind of sexual behavior we indulge in or the sex of the person we choose as a partner."[10]

It seems that the common thread among people who have become homosexuals is an unhealthy relationship between them and their parents. Although not every home where there is a dominant mother and a weak, poor role model for a father will produce a homosexual son, many homosexuals have that kind of home. Homosexuals also generally tell about being used by a homosexual for sex early in puberty or even before. Because they were enticed into such acts a number of times and found it pleasurable, they became hooked on it much as a smoker gets hooked on nicotine.

Some researchers believe there are genetic reasons people become homosexuals.[11] Recently uncovered evidence indicates that genes may be at least part of the reason some people become alcoholics. But even if a person's genes might encourage him toward alcoholism, that doesn't mean that he can't overcome that temptation. The same would be true of homosexuals.

Fear of Being Homosexual

One of the fears I had during part of my high school years was that I might discover that I was homosexual. I remember the day I got up enough courage to share with my mother (we could usually talk about almost anything) how that frightened me. I was relieved by her answer.

It's common for young people, especially boys, to be troubled about the possibility of becoming homosexual. Sometimes that fear is the result of having been approached for homosexual sex. Other times the fear comes from being acquainted with someone who is homosexual, a friend or relative. Young people might even be afraid because they are very close friends with someone of the same gender. And there are times when adolescents worry about being homosexual because they participated in same-sex sexual exploration or play, perhaps even reaching orgasm. But those are not reasons to fear that one might be or become homosexual.

On one of our anniversaries, when I took my wife out to eat, I left her standing on a street corner while I walked the block and a half to get the car. When I picked her up, she jumped into the car more quickly than I expected she would. Her face was flushed. It took her several minutes to regain her composure. Then she told me how a man had approached her for sex while she was waiting for me. Now think about that. The fact that someone asked my wife for sex doesn't make her a prostitute, does it? And if someone of your gender asks you for sex, that doesn't make you a homosexual.

Having a friend or relative who is a homosexual doesn't make a person homosexual either. Having a friend who is overweight will not make you overweight. Having a friend who is thin will not make you thin. Having a friend who is homosexual will not make you homosexual. However, as with all our friends, we always have to be aware of how much influence they are having on us and whether that influence is positive or negative.

It is also not unnatural for a teenager to have a deep attachment for someone of his/her gender. That person may be another teen or a favorite teacher or friend of the family. God uses such admiration to help us sort out the kind of person he wants us to be and the direction he wants us to take in our lives. Don't allow fear of homosexuality to deprive you of a close association with your father if you are a boy or with your mother if you are a girl. That definitely includes giving and receiving hugs from them.

Feeling Accused

Satan often reminds Christian teens of their sexual sins. He's not called "The Accuser" for nothing. He works best when he can get us to doubt that all our sins have been completely forgiven by Jesus. Some of those doubts are raised because it is not uncommon for a teen to have been part of some kind of sex play with members of his/her gender. Satan tries hard to convince believing young people that such activity means they are homosexual or at least very abnormal.

The fact is, although such sex play is sinful, normal young people are often involved in it, and it has no bearing on their future sexual preferences. One study of twelve-year-old boys found that four out of ten (39%) had joined in such sex play. Fourteen percent of nine-year-old girls had as well.[12] It is also common for young teens to feel sexually excited around members of their gender and to become aroused by pornographic pictures of people of their own sex.

It may take a long time for a person to feel at ease with members of the opposite sex. The fact that a person has not felt the need to date during high school doesn't make him a homosexual. And a person is certainly not homosexual because he has not had heterosexual sex. One should become concerned about his sexual orientation only when, as an adult, he/she continually experiences sexual interest in members of the same gender. If that is the case, the person should talk with his parents, his pastor, or a Christian counselor.

If you are feeling uneasy about the thought of being a homosexual, give yourself time. Those fears are rather common. As you grow and mature, they will probably disappear. But I also want you to know that you are not the only one who is afraid of being rejected, who is scared about being with someone of the opposite sex, and who is insecure. There's a lot of that around. You are normal. Continue to pray for the Lord to help you overcome those negative feelings. But you also need to know this: he might answer your prayer by putting you in a situation where you will be forced to get to know some folks of the opposite gender and by teaching you how to face your fears.

God's View

God does not consider homosexuality an "alternate lifestyle" that is just as acceptable as the heterosexual lifestyle. God calls homosexuality a sin.

Homosexuality is mentioned seven times in the Bible, never in positive terms. You might want to look up those passages for yourself. They are Genesis 19:1-11; Leviticus 18:22; 20:13; Judges 19:22-25; Romans 1:26,27; 1 Corinthians 6:9,10; and 1 Timothy 1:9,10. 1 Corinthians 6:9,10 is very clear about the way God looks at homosexuality:

> Do you not know that the wicked will not inherit the kingdom of God? Do not be deceived: Neither the sexually immoral nor idolaters nor adulterers nor male prostitutes nor homosexual offenders nor thieves nor the greedy nor drunkards nor slanderers nor swindlers will inherit the kingdom of God.

The Romans passage is of special interest because God says that homosexuality is the result of turning one's back on the Lord. It shouldn't surprise us, then, to hear growing support for homosexual lifestyles the more our country gets away from Christianity. That passage says,

> For although they knew God, they neither glorified him as God nor gave thanks to him, but their thinking became futile and their foolish hearts were darkened....

> Therefore God gave them over in the sinful desires of their hearts to sexual impurity for the degrading of their bodies with one another. They exchanged the truth of God for a lie, and worshiped and served created things rather than the Creator—who is forever praised. Amen.

> Because of this, God gave them over to shameful lusts. Even their women exchanged natural relations for unnatural ones. In the same way the men also abandoned natural relations with women and were inflamed with lust for one another. Men committed indecent acts with other men, and received in themselves the due penalty for their perversion (verses 21, 24-27).

Homosexuality does not fit God's command to Adam and Eve, "Be fruitful and increase in number." Homosexuality won't allow God's purpose for making us sexual creatures to be accomplished. Doesn't it seem to you that, if homosexual relationships were what God intended, he would have created Adam and Andy rather than Adam and Eve?

At the same time, we need to be reminded that Jesus died for the sins of homosexuals as much as he died to forgive any one of us. The passage from 1 Corinthians you just read has a wonderful verse right after it: "And that is what some of you were [homosexuals, idolaters, alcoholics, etc.]. But you were washed, you were sanctified [made holy], you were justified [declared not guilty] in the name of the Lord Jesus Christ and by the Spirit of our God."

Jesus' resurrection has guaranteed forgiveness to homosexuals and anyone who is involved in any kind of sexual perversion. That forgiveness is ours for the believing. And as a person believes it, he will want to thank God for his forgiveness by giving up the sins in his life and working to keep those sins away. That's repentance.

Helping

Christians will agree with their Father about homosexuality. They cannot say it's OK when God has said it is not. But Christians will also be as concerned about homosexuals as their Father is. He loves them. He's loved them enough to punish his Son for their sins. He forgives them as they trust in Jesus as their Savior. Christians, too, will love, help, and forgive homosexuals.

We'll certainly avoid making fun of anyone by accusing him/her of that sin. Gossiping about people, spreading rumors that they might be homosexuals, is outside the Christian lifestyle. Even if we know for certain that someone is a homosexual, that does not give us the right to tease him, mock him, and ruin his reputation. Slang names like queer, fag, homo, fairy, queen, fruit shouldn't even be part of our vocabulary according to Ephesians 4:29: "Do not let any unwholesome talk come out of your mouths, but only what is helpful for building others up according to their needs, that it may benefit those who listen."

A homosexual may always have the desire for same-sex sex, and that desire is sinful in itself, but the sin is compounded when he/she hangs on to those sinful thoughts and acts on them. The good news is that those homosexual desires do not need to be acted on any more than heterosexual desires need to be acted on.

But suppose that the Lord puts you in contact with a classmate who is homosexual. What might you do to help him/her?

First, you need to know that homosexuality is not a sickness that can be "cured." Homosexuality is not even something that a person is. It is something a person does. Homosexuality is an activity, a habit, a lifestyle that can be changed. It is possible to develop new ways of relating to others on a sexual level. We heard Paul say there were homosexuals in the Corinthian congregation, but they were empowered by God to change ("such *were* some of you"). Whether a person will give up his homosexual practices or not depends much on his willingness to conform to what God wants.

So what should you do if you suspect a friend is homosexual?

1. You certainly need to start praying for him—and don't stop. Pray especially that he would come to believe in Jesus and grow in that faith. Pray that any hold Satan has in his life would be broken.

2. Then keep building your relationship with him/her so he/she trusts you and is willing to confide in you. Chances are he/she is quite lonely inside because of that secret.

3. Be open for an opportunity to talk about sexuality, and be willing to listen. That doesn't mean that you have to agree with what your friend believes. Listening means just that: listening. Please remember: at this point quoting a bunch of Bible passages to condemn your friend would not be helpful.

4. If your friend thinks that he/she is homosexual, you might want to lend him/her this book and suggest he/she reads this chapter.

5. Talk about how knowing Jesus is your Savior helps you deal with sexual sins and how he has given you the power to conquer sin in a number of areas. Share how appreciative you are that he has forgiven you and given you heaven.

6. Encourage your friend to break off any relationships he/she has with other homosexuals. Perhaps there is a Christian support group of other people who are dealing with overcoming their homosexuality he/she could join. Ask your pastor or counselor at school. Be careful though. Some support groups try to help people become more comfortable with being homosexual. Try to help your friend find new Christian friends who will be a positive influence on him/her.

7. Keep being a friend. The only time you should back away is if your friend's negative influence on you is greater than your positive influence on him/her. But then that's good advice for any friendship. In the meanwhile, don't stop showing you care about him/her as a friend because you are a Christian, and keep working on the first six

steps. One does not become a homosexual overnight. Without a miracle, one will not stop being a homosexual overnight either.

A Way to Say Thanks

I lost track of Roger some years ago. I fear for his health. I know that he traveled quite widely, spending time in the homosexual communities of New York City and San Francisco.

Like all sin, homosexuality carries with it its own earthly punishment. It's no wonder God warns us to stay away from it. He loves us too much to let us hurt ourselves without at least shouting out to us, "Don't do that! You'll get in trouble!"

And now he gives us an opportunity to be his lips and to warn people around us, "Watch out! That's dangerous!" I want to be used by God to do that because he has made me his child and promised me eternal life with him. Warning others about sin and telling them about Jesus is a way I can thank God for warning me and telling me about his Son. It's a way you can thank God, too.

Dear Father, thank you for the assurance you gave me about my sexuality in this chapter. There have been times I've wondered whether I might be a homosexual. Thank you, too, for reminding me that homosexuality is a sin that Jesus has forgiven along with all other sins. Help me to have loving attitudes toward people who practice that lifestyle. Use me to minister

to them in whatever way you have prepared me to do so.

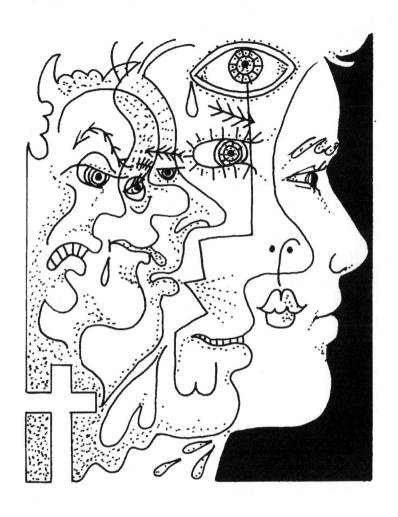

15.

SEX THAT PERVERTS

When I was growing up, I remember being warned about an older boy who lived on my block. Donny was kind of a weird kid anyway. He scared me just because of the way he acted around smaller kids like me and my friends. But when my mother sternly told me never to allow Donny to pull down my pants and touch me, I knew that he was one person I didn't want anything to do with.

People weren't as open about deviant sexual behavior when I was small as they are today. That's why my little town put up with Donny as long as it did.

The society we share knows more about sexual behavior that is not normal and has much better laws against it. We also have better treatment programs for those who are driven by such behavior.

Deviant Sex

Sexual practices which deviate from normal, moral forms of expressing ourselves sexually are deviant sex. Sometimes these practices are called perversions, and people who practice them are said to be perverted. Those who enjoy deviant sex have psychological and spiritual problems which require professional help.

But please remember: just as God has loved and sent his Son for homosexuals, he has loved and sent his Son for those who practice other forms of sexual perversion. We, too, as people who are thankful for God's goodness, will want to love those whose problems have led them into such sins.

Types of Deviations

Some men obtain sexual satisfaction from showing

their genitals to others. They are called **exhibition-ists** or flashers. Exhibitionists usually expose themselves to young girls. They enjoy seeing how shocked their victims are.

Voyeurs find sexual stimulation in watching others have sex or watching others who are in some degree of being undressed. Voyeurs are also called "peeping toms" because they may "peep" (look) into bedroom windows at night to see what is happening there. Sometimes they are caught by the police and arrested for that.

Some people have a **fetish** for an item they find sexually arousing. Everyone finds some things to be especially sexually stimulating. For some it may be certain body parts of the opposite sex (breasts, hair, muscles). For others it may be a piece of clothing (shoes, underwear, a blouse) or an odor (perfume, perspiration). That is normal. A person with a fetish, however, isn't just aroused by that thing. Whatever arouses him becomes a compulsion (an urge that seems irresistible). That article becomes his "loved one" and actually takes the place of a human sexual partner. Other forms of fetishism include **kleptomania**, stealing things of no value to the person for the sexual high it gives him/her and **pyromania**, setting fires and watching them burn for the sexual excitement it offers him/her.

Women with uncontrollable sexual desires which cause them to seek sexual intercourse with anyone at any cost are called **nymphomaniacs**. This is a very rare form of mental illness.

Pedophilia is the compulsion to have sex with children. My teenage neighbor Donny was a pedophile.

Sadists and masochists are people who link sex with violence. For the sadist, sexual pleasure comes with giving pain. Masochists find they receive the most pleasure during sex if it is painful. Sometimes these sexual deviations are called "S and M" for sadism and masochism.

Necrophilia is the desire to have sex with a corpse. Bestiality is having sex with an animal.

A **prostitute** is someone who agrees to sexual activity with another in return for money, drugs, or other items of value. Prostitutes may be male or female and may engage in heterosexual or homosexual sex. Prostitutes are very much at risk for contracting sexually transmitted diseases. Thousands of prostitutes, along with their sexual partners (called "johns") are arrested each year.

Another form of sexual deviation is **seduction**. When someone is gently enticed into sexual activity, even though that person doesn't want sex, he/she is seduced. Seduction can happen in heterosexual and homosexual relationships. Some men seduce their girlfriends by telling their dates how much they love them, how beautiful they are, how important those dates are to them. Those women feel crushed and foolish when they find out that their boyfriend was only using them to satisfy his own sex drive.

Incest is also a form of sexual deviation. We speak about that in the next chapter.

Pornography

People who regularly view pornography are also

caught in deviant sexual activity. Pornography may portray normal sexual relations between men and women. It may also include pictures or films of the sexual activity you've just read about. That means most of the R-rated movies contain pornographic scenes.

Pornography feeds our minds powerful messages about what some people think sex is really like. And the messages we receive there are much different from what God tells us. Pictures of naked bodies in suggestive poses say, "Sex is a plaything. Use it any way you please. Just have fun." Those pictures tell us, "Women are to be used to satisfy men's sexual desires. They are not really people. They are things."

Pornography pollutes our minds just as toxic waste pollutes rivers and lakes. It feeds lust. It encourages us to think of the person pictured there as a sex object rather than as a person who needs our love, support, and care. Pornography robs us of seeing other humans for the beautiful art forms God has made them. And worse yet, once we watch pornography, those images are stored away in our minds and are easily called up and reviewed by lust.

Read the end of the chapter called "Solo Sex" for some suggestions on overcoming lust in your life.

Rape

Rape is one person forcing another person to have sex. It can be committed by either sex against members of either sex. Although we may think that rape is mostly a crime against women, more and more men are being raped too.

Rape is an act of violence, not lust. The rapist is a person who is angry to an unhealthy degree and expresses his rage through sexually dominating another person. The rapist is not as interested in satisfying his sex drive as he is in controlling the person he rapes by hurting and frightening her. Most often, the person who is raped knows his/her attacker.

"Date rape" happens when one's date forces him/her to have sex or to go further sexually than he/she wants to go. "Date rape" is against the law. You have the right to say "no" to your date regardless of how much money he/she has spent on you or how far you have allowed your situation to go sexually. The law says that your date must respect your wishes. It is against the law for anyone to force you to have sex.

What should you do if you are raped? Go immediately to a hospital or rape crisis center. There will be people there who are trained to help. They will be understanding and sympathetic. A doctor will check you for injuries. Sperm cells will be collected to be used as evidence against the rapist. For that reason, you should not shower or wash before going to the hospital. The doctor will also take steps to prevent you from becoming infected with a STD. The hospital will recommend a way for you to receive counseling so that you can deal with your experience. You will want to seek out that kind of help. It's also a very good idea to speak with your pastor.

The best defense against rape is to stay away from situations where you put yourself in danger of being attacked. Walking alone at night and hitchhiking can invite rapists to make you their victim. Many women carry a whistle they can blow to summon help if they find themselves in danger. It is also a good idea never to go out alone with a person you have just met or don't really know. Never allow yourself to be "picked up" at a dance or on a street. And, of course, it makes sense not to flirt with someone you don't know.

The Christian Response to Deviation

It's easy for us to turn away from people who are caught up in sins of sexual deviation. What they do seems to us to be sick and unsavory. And it is. It is not normal. It is sinful.

Because we are the children of the God of light, we'll not want to put ourselves in a position where we'll be tempted to become involved in those sins. Staying away from those who are involved will be helpful in keeping ourselves safe.

But we don't show Jesus' kind of love to people who practice deviant sex by turning our backs on them, either. They, too, need to hear about the forgiveness Jesus has won for everyone. They need to know that there are people in our churches who can help them and support them in overcoming their sin. They need to know that in our Christian communities they will not be ridiculed. After all, their sin is not any worse in God's eyes than any of our sins—and God has forgiven us all our sins. They need to know of the great victory that Jesus has won for us that gives us not only eternal life, but also the power to live full and free lives here.

Our loving heavenly Father, there are so many ways to misuse your precious gift of human sexuality. Sometimes we are responsible for misusing that gift. Forgive us and help us to love you better so that we use your gift as we should. We ask that you would work powerfully in the lives of everyone who is guilty of deviant sex. Lead them to freedom as you bring them to a close relationship with Jesus. We dare to ask for this blessing because Jesus is our Savior.

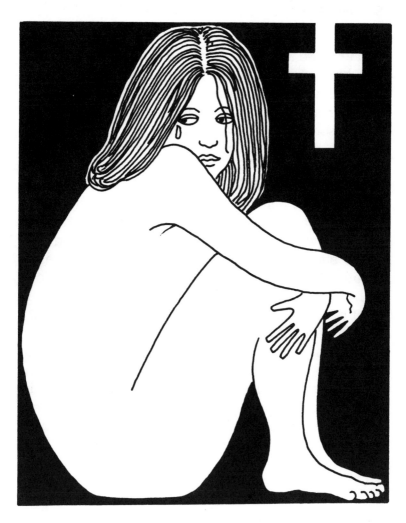

16.

SEX THAT HURTS

"He made me take my clothes off and get into bed with him."

After months of working with Sheila so she would trust me, she was finally sharing the heart of her pain, the reason for her low self-worth, the force that led her into drugs and alcohol, and the thing that kept shoving her toward suicide. She told a sad, sad story about herself as a little six-year-old girl who was sexually abused by her father. She described a mother who either didn't want to admit her husband would do that or didn't want to be bothered. She cried when she spoke about her mother telling her she was "crazy" because "your father would never do that." She told of her parents making her swear she would conceal what was happening and the heavy burden she had to carry because of that terrible secret.

Sheila is a combination of people I've gotten to know—both men and women. Their stories, though different, are similar. They each tried to live with their terrible secret always gnawing at them. They blamed themselves for causing their abuse. They saw themselves as wicked, unlovable people who were not worth anything.

Chances are you know someone like Sheila. Perhaps you are someone like Sheila. One study of children and teenagers found that one in four teenage girls was sexually molested at least once in her life.[13]

In this chapter we're going to talk about how God's gift of sex is perverted by sexual activity within families. If you are someone who has been the victim of this kind of abuse, I want you to know that there are people in your life who will understand, who will believe you, and who want to help. Even more important, I want you to know you are loved. God loves you. He accepts you. He wants to use even that terrible experience to benefit you. Please read on.

Incest

Sexual intercourse between family members is called incest. Every state has some kind of law against incest. Although laws vary from state to state, many prohibit marriage or sexual contact not only between parents and children and brothers and sisters, but between first and second cousins. One of the reasons for this is genetic. A high rate of deformed or handicapped children results from incestuous relationships. An even more powerful reason is the psychological harm that incest causes in the lives of the people who are victims of incest.

God made it clear to his Old Testament people that incest was contrary to his will. Leviticus 18:6-18 lists all the kinds of sexual relations within a family that are not moral:

No one is to approach any close relative to have sexual relations. I am the Lord. Do not dishonor your father by having sexual relations with your mother. She is your mother; do not have relations with her. Do not have sexual relations with your father's wife; that would dishonor your father. Do not have sexual relations with your sister, either your father's daughter or your mother's daughter, whether she was born in the same home or elsewhere. Do not have sexual relations with your son's daughter or your daughter's daughter; that would dishonor you. Do not have sexual relations with the daughter of your father's wife, born to your father; she is your sister. Do not have sexual relations with your father's sister; she is your father's close relative. Do not have sexual relations with your mother's sister, because she is your mother's close relative. Do not dishonor your father's brother by approaching his wife to have sexual relations; she is your aunt. Do not have sexual relations with your daughter-in-law. She is your son's wife; do not have relations with her. Do not have sexual relations with your brother's wife; that would dishonor your brother. Do not have sexual relations with both a woman and her daughter. Do not have sexual relations with either her son's daughter or her daughter's daughter; they are her close relatives. That is wickedness. Do not take your wife's sister as a rival wife and have sexual relations with her while your wife is living.

Also check Deuteronomy 22:30.

In the New Testament Paul insisted that the Corinthian congregation excommunicate a man who was living with his father's wife (perhaps his father had remarried and then died, since the woman is not called the man's mother). Because the man was not repentant and refused to give up the relationship, Paul maintained that he showed he was not a Christian. Read about that in 1 Corinthians 5.

Even though incest is not considered right by our government or God, it still happens. And it happens frequently. Incest takes place in families that are upper class, middle class, and lower class. Families of every race are affected by it.

Young children of the same family may satisfy their natural curiosity about the opposite sex with each other. This is not actually incest.

True incest often involves an older relative (a father, uncle, cousin, or a person close to the family). That person may force himself or herself on the victim or gently seduce his victim into having sex. The abuser usually threatens to hurt his victim if she tells. He may assure her, "You are special. We have a relationship that no one will understand. If you tell, your mother (or sisters, etc.) will be jealous. We need to keep this little secret to ourselves." He may use guilt feelings to keep her from telling. "I couldn't control myself. You made me have sex with you." Or "If you tell, the police will come to arrest me. It will be your fault if I go to jail."

The Sexually Abused

In most cases, people who sexually abuse others were sexually abused themselves when they were children. They might not even remember their own abuse because they have blocked it out of their minds. No one knows why people who were sexually abused as children tend to abuse children when they get older, but it usually works that way. That is one reason people who have been sexually abused as children or teens need to seek counseling.

Those who have been sexually abused may also become sexually active, even promiscuous. Sexual abuse victims may use sexual activity as a way to try to feel good about themselves. Their experience with sexual abuse may make them feel worthless. To make themselves feel worth something, they say yes to sex. They think that, if they are sexually active, other people will love them and accept them. Unfortunately, promiscuous sexual activity only makes people feel used and leads them to feel worse about themselves.

If You're a Victim

People who have been sexually abused by family members or friends of the family need to know that they are not guilty. **Please listen to this**. If you have been used by someone for incest, it is not your fault. You have nothing to feel guilty about. Do not blame yourself. Refuse to allow yourself to think that you are not worth anything or that you are now ruined as a person.

When God sent Jesus to be the Savior, Jesus atoned for all sins to all people for all times. Jesus "is the atoning sacrifice for our sins, and not only for ours but also for the sins of the whole world" (1 John 2:2). There is no way that Jesus hasn't made you right with God, no matter what wrong things you have done or think you have done. The fact is that God has forgiven and accepted as his own dear child the worst sinner of all, so he has to have forgiven and accepted you, too. Don't you remember how Paul said, "Here is a trustworthy saying that deserves full acceptance: Christ Jesus came into the world to save sinners—of whom I am the worst"? (1 Timothy 1:15).

And there's more good news. Not only does God want to be close to you, God wants to use what you have been through to make you more effective in serving him. In the verse that follows the one you just read, Paul says, "I was shown mercy so that in me, the worst of sinners, Christ Jesus might display his unlimited patience as an example for those who would believe on him and receive eternal life" (1 Timothy 1:16).

A To-Do List

Here are some things I'd like you to do if you have been abused by someone in your family or a friend of your family or anyone else. And, please be aware that abuse doesn't just mean being forced or fooled into having sex. Any improper touching or even talking about sexual matters with you is sexual abuse.

1. Tell someone. That's probably going to be hard. It's not easy to tell others about being sexually abused. But you need someone to help you think through what has been happening to you. No one can come through being sexually abused without needing help. Tell someone. The person you go to might be your pastor, a counselor at school, a teacher you feel you can trust, your doctor, or an agency in your area especially designed to help people in your situation (it may be called something like "Task Force on Sexual Assault and Domestic Abuse").

   If you keep your abuse to yourself, you may be putting other people in danger. Abusers rarely hurt just one person. They normally have a long track record of forcing themselves on others. The person who is abusing you has probably abused (or will abuse) your sisters/brothers, cousins, and even neighborhood children.

2. Keep telling people until you find help. Sometimes when a person who has been sexually abused tells what has happened, he/she is not believed. My friend Sheila had a mother who would not believe her. If that happens to you, do not give up trying to tell someone. Keep on telling people until you find someone who will believe you and offer to help.

3. When the person who is abusing you approaches you for sex, resist his advances by making it clear to him that you will tell others about what he is doing. If he does not leave you alone, carry out your threat. Do not allow this person to threaten you, persuade you, or make you feel so guilty that you will not tell. What is happening to you is not good for you. There is no such thing as a positive incestuous relationship.

Don't Forget

If you have been a victim of incest, you need to remember you are still a valuable, important person. If you have a friend who is an incest victim, he/she needs to know that, too. And here's the thing that makes you valuable and important: "The blood of Jesus, [God's] Son, purifies us from all sin" (1 John 1:7), even those sins others commit against us. Because Jesus makes sure you are looked at by God as "pure," you can be sure God's promises are yours:

The righteous will shine like the sun in the kingdom of their Father (Matthew 13:43).

You are a chosen people, a royal priesthood, a holy nation, a people belonging to God, that you may declare the praises of him who called you out of darkness into his wonderful light. Once you were not a people, but now you are the people of God; once you had not received mercy, but now you have received mercy (1 Peter 2:9,10).

God wants to assure you of his love and acceptance. He wants to help you. But he's probably going to supply that assistance through another human being. Find that someone he has in mind to help you deal with what you've been through.

Dear Father in heaven, our hearts break to think of the many young people who have had to suffer sexual abuse. You never intended your wonderful gift of sex to be used like that. We pray for them, asking you to give them the strength to trust you more, to claim your promises of love and acceptance, and to find the person you have prepared to help them deal with their situation. Protect them, Father. Help them to know what real love is. Enable them to live like the chosen people, royal priesthood, holy nation, and people who belong to you that they are because of Jesus.

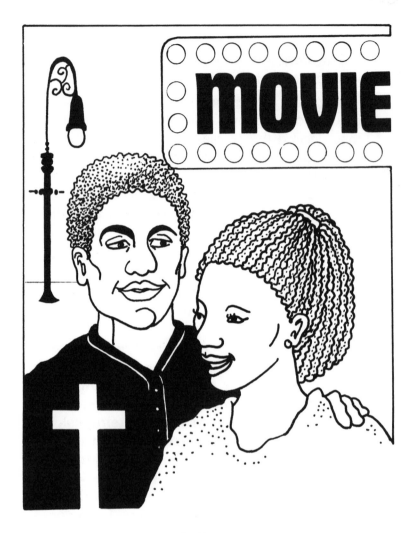

17.

GOD, THANK YOU I'M SEXUAL

I walked her home after a movie. I and about a half dozen of her friends.

In the little village of 2,000 people where I grew up in northern Wisconsin there was one movie theater. Sometimes the movies made it to the television screen before they made it to the theater screen. But every Friday night kids from all over town turned out for whatever was playing. Of course, back then every movie was G-rated, so Friday after Friday found my friends and me taking in a movie, sometimes a double feature.

About eighth grade, though, the group of guys I hung around with began to notice that there were groups of girls who were also going to the movies. Then we started sitting behind them—just to tease and be weird, at least until the usher came down the aisle and threatened to show us out the door.

Several Friday nights later, the next step was for one of the guys to sit next to one of the girls. I was elected. Maybe I volunteered. I can't remember. At any rate, urged on by my buddies, I ended up sitting next to Alicia, who was surrounded by her covey of friends.

That was brave stuff. My heart pounded. I didn't know what to say. In my embarrassment all sorts of silly things came out of my mouth ("Alicia, do you come here often?" "Your friends are really strange.") And all the while her friends twittered away, as my friends who were sitting behind us hooted.

The guys teased me the next week. "Jim sat with Alicia!" they chanted. I found out later their song wasn't so much to put me down as it was to cover their own lack of courage. They were wishing they had been brave enough to sit next to Alicia.

I didn't appreciate their teasing. I might even have threatened a couple of them with physical harm if they kept it up. But I found out that sitting next to a girl from my class at the movie was worth the hard time the guys gave me. It was a grand experience. I felt excited, scared, grown up, dumb, nervous, exhilarated, and many other things all at the same time and all mixed up.

A few more weeks down the road, I even walked Alicia (and her bodyguard of friends) home after a movie. The guys tagged along at a comfortable distance. They lobbed catcalls as we went and made something of a scene.

It's funny, though. Three years later almost every one of my friends was dating and thought nothing of walking their girlfriends home after a movie. Still not all of my friends were comfortable being with a girl. Some didn't start dating until after high school. But at least, as they got older, they didn't keep making strange noises and following around those of us who were dating.

Girl/boy relationships are going to be different for everyone. Some of your friends probably will be more interested in the opposite sex than you. Some probably will be less interested. That's OK. Take it at your own speed. There is not just one right way to develop physically or socially through your teen years.

Many things will confuse you in your transition from child to adult. It's that way for everyone. Don't be afraid to admit that. If your friends deny it, they're not being honest with you. Even the teens you know who seem to have it all together have wrestled with the same things you are wrestling with—maybe not at the same time as you or in the same way, but they've wrestled with them.

More than anything, though, you're going to need a close knowledgeable friend to help you sort things out from time to time. Someone close to your age will be helpful if he/she is a Christian and has his/her relationship with Jesus on good terms. Your parents can be a help, but you'll both have to work on keeping lines of communication open. Books like this will help, too.

But there's one friend who will help more than all the rest. The friend who loved you enough to die for you. The friend who has promised, "I am the good shepherd. The good shepherd lays down his life for the sheep. . . . I give them eternal life, and they shall never perish; no one can snatch them out of my hand" (John 10:11,28). He will be there to help you as he speaks to you through his word, as you commune regularly, as you worship, as you do Bible study with others. And you will be blessed as you not only listen to him speak to you, but also act on what he says. You know his promise, "Blessed . . . are those who hear the word of God and obey it" (Luke 11:28).

Jesus is the friend who has enabled you to be a dearly loved child of the God of the universe. Jesus is the friend who stands by you to provide for you, protect you, guide you, and care for you as long as you live here. Jesus is the friend who will meet you with a big smile and open arms at heaven's gates when you die and welcome you in. Jesus is just the friend you need as you take your place in his world as an adult.

Jesus, thanks for being my friend. There are a lot of things I find hard to talk about with others, even my closest friends. But I know you'll always be there for me. You'll listen to me, even when I just jabber on. You'll direct me whenever I listen to your word. And I know I can always trust your advice. What you went through on the cross proves that. I feel so secure knowing you're there for me.

Help me take full advantage of your friendship. Keep me committed to talking with you each day. And lead me to dig into your word. Most of all, help me to keep marveling about your love for me so I dedicate everything I am to you and face the facts about who you have made me with excitement and joy.

ENDNOTES

1. (page 27) The Statistical Abstract of the United States 1990 shows how women have caught up to men in levels of education (Table 274). In 1987 men and women earned equal numbers of college and post graduate degrees. The Abstract also exhibits that women earn from 1/3 to 1/2 of men's income (Tables 731, 737). "Trouble at the Top," *US News and World Report* (06/17/91, pages 40-48) reports that "'a glass ceiling' blocks women from corporate heights."

2. (page 52) Further reading on human conception and development during pregnancy may include:

   The Gift of Sex, Clifford and Joyce Penner, Word, 1983.

   Handbook on Abortion, Dr. and Mrs J.C. Wilke, Hayes, 1975.

   Love, Sex, and God, Bill Ameiss and Jane Graver, Concordia, 1988.

   Parent's Guide to Sex Education, Mary Ann Mayo, Zondervan, 1986.

   Sex Education Is for the Family, Tim LaHaye, Zondervan, 1985.

3. (page 32) Further reading on the male reproductive system may include:

   The Gift of Sex, Clifford and Joyce Penner, Word, 1983.

   Love, Sex, and God, Bill Ameiss and Jane Graver, Concordia, 1988.

   Parent's Guide to Sex Education, Mary Ann Mayo, Zondervan, 1986.

Sex Education Is for the Family, Tim LaHaye, Zondervan, 1985.

4. (page 37) Further reading on the female reproductive system may include:

The Gift of Sex, Clifford and Joyce Penner, Word, 1983.

Love, Sex, and God, Bill Ameiss and Jane Graver, Concordia, 1988.

Parent's Guide to Sex Education, Mary Ann Mayo, Zondervan, 1986.

Sex Education Is for the Family, Tim LaHaye, Zondervan, 1985.

5. (page 46) For current statistics about the impact of STDs in the United States contact the National Centers for Disease Control at 1-800-227-8922.

6. (page 46) *The Milwaukee Journal* (08/14/90, B-1) reported, "There have been 227 cases of syphilis reported in Milwaukee in the first six months of this year, a pace that is expected to produce 454 cases this year, or more than double the 212 cases reported last year." *The Milwaukee Journal* reported on December 15, 1991 that the total syphilis cases in the city for the first ten months of the year stood at 678. The National Centers for Disease Control in Atlanta reported that "the number of syphilis cases hit a 40-year high (in 1989). . . . The estimated 44,000 cases of potentially deadly venereal disease in 1989 represents a 56 percent increase from the number of cases in 1986, said Dr. Ward Cates, head of the sexually transmitted disease division" (reported in the *Daily Herald*, Northwest Suburban Chicago, 02/02/90).

7. (page 107) Researchers Mark D. Haward and Junichi Yagi, "Contraceptive Failure in the United States: Estimates from the 1982 National Survey of Family Growth," Table 5. Researchers Melvin Zelnik, Michael A.K. Koenig, and Kim Young. "Sources of Prescription Contraceptives and Subsequent Pregnancy among Young Women." Family Planning Perspectives: January/February, 1984.

8. (page 62) Researchers Mark D. Haward and Junichi Yagi,

"Contraceptive Failure in the United States: Estimates from the 1982 National Survey of Family Growth," Table 5. Researchers Melvin Zelnik, Michael A.K. Koenig, and Kim Young. "Sources of Prescription Contraceptives and Subsequent Pregnancy among Young Women." Family Planning Perspectives: January/February, 1984.

9. (page 107) *The Chicago Sun Times* (May 5, 1989) quoted a study that appeared in *Lancet*, a British medical journal. It said, "Young women who take contraceptive pills for four years or more run an increased risk of developing breast cancer, according to a five year study which is the largest of its kind focused on British women under 36. It said four to eight years on popular brands of the Pill increased the risk of breast cancer by 40 percent while more than eight years increased the risk by about 70 percent."

10. (page 75) *Eros Defiled*, John White, Inter-Varsity Press, 1977, page 116.

11. (page 75) The December 15, 1991 *Milwaukee Journal* (page A 16) quoted an AP article, dateline Chicago, which said, "A study of twins suggests that homosexuality has a genetic or biological basis. . . . 'We found 52% of identical twin brothers of gay men also were gay, compared with 22% of fraternal twins, compared with 11% of genetically unrelated (adoptive) brothers,' said J. Michael Bailey, assistant professor of psychology at Northwestern University in Evanston."

12. (page 76) "Parents' Guide to Sex Education," Mary Ann Mayo, Zondervan, 1986, page 148.

13. (page 86) James McCary (*Human Sexuality,* page 377) cites a Kinsey group survey which found that 20-25% of 4-13 year old girls had been approached for sex and 35% of college age women who had "some form of experience during childhood with sexual variants" (most of whom were exhibitionists). Tim LaHaye in *Sex Education Is for the Family* (page 115) refers to a survey of 800 college students. Nineteen percent of the females and nine percent of the males indicated they had been sexually abused as children. Alvin Rosenbaum in *The Young People's Yellow*

Pages (Perigee Books, 1983) notes that one percent of women have been sexually molested as children by their fathers or step-fathers.

BIBLIOGRAPHY

AIDS and Young People, Robert Redfield and Wanda Kay Franz, Regnery Gateway, 1987.

Christian Living in the Home, Jay E. Adams, Baker, 1972.

Eros Defiled, John White, Inter-Varsity Press, 1977.

From Teens to Marriage, Reuben D. Behlmer, Concordia, 1962.

The Gift of Sex, Clifford and Joyce Penner, Word, 1983.

Handbook on Abortion, Dr. and Mrs. J.C. Wilke, Hayes, 1975.

Handling Your Hormones, Jim Burns, Merit Books, 1984.

How to Help Your Child Say No to Sexual Pressure (book and video) Josh McDowell, Word, 1987.

How to Really Love Your Child, Dr. Ross Campbell, Victor Books, 1989.

Human Sexuality, James Leslie McCary, D.Van Nostrand Co., 1973.

I-Questions God Answers Course 3, James A. Aderman and Paul E. Kelm, Northwetsern Publishing House, 1991.

The Key to Your Child's Heart, Gary Smalley, Word, 1984.

Let's Talk About Love and Sex (video), Josh McDowell, Word, 1988.

Life Can Be Sexual, Elmer N. Witt, Concordia, 1967.

Living in Grace, Wisconsin Lutheran Child and Family Service, 1976.

Love, Dad, Josh McDowell, Word, 1988.

Love, Sex, and God, Bill Ameiss and Jane Graver, Concordia, 1988.

The Next Time I Fall in Love, Chap Clark, Zondervan, 1987.

No Second Chance (video), Jeremiah Films, 1991.

Parent's Guide to Sex Education, Mary Ann Mayo, Zondervan, 1986.

Questions Teenagers Ask About Dating and Sex, Barry Wood, Revell, 1981.

Sex Education Is for the Family, Tim LaHaye, Zondervan, 1985.Sex Respect: the Option of True Sexual Freedom, Coleen Kelly Mast, 1986.

Sex without Fear, S.A. Lewin and John Gilmore, Medical Research Press, fourth revised edition, 1975.

Sexuality and Dating, Richard Reichert, St. Mary Press, 1981.

Statistical Abstract of the United States 1990, U.S. Department of Commerce, 1990.

Teaching True Abstinence Sex Education, Pat Socia, Project Respect, 1990.

What I Wish Somebody Had Told Me About Sex When I Was Thirteen, Stephen M. Crotts, Fairway, 1987.

INDEX

Abortifacients, 104, 106, 111

Abortion, 44, 106-107, 163, 167

Acne, 2, 87, 89, 116

Adolescence, 2-6, 8, 86, 117-118

Adolescent, 2, 59, 89, 120

AIDS, 80-83, 129, 167

Amniotic fluid, 43-44, 50

Athletic supporter, 60

Autoeroticism, 94

Bestiality, 144

Birth canal, 50, 65

Birth control, 104, 106-107, 111

Birth defects, 46-48, 81

Bladder, 57, 66

Bladder infection, 66

Blastocyst, 46

Blue balls, 60

Breast, 67-68, 74-75, 87-88, 108, 143, 165

Cervix, 40, 50, 58, 65, 105-106

Chromosomes, 41, 49, 52

Circumcision, 58

Clitoris, 67

Conception, 40-44, 47, 72, 104-108, 163

Condom, 82-83, 104-105, 108

Contraceptive, 22, 104-105, 108-112, 164-165

Cowper's gland, 57

Cramps, 49-50, 65, 74, 76

Date rape, 146

Deviations, 142, 144. *See also* Sexual deviation

Diaphragm, 105

Douche, 66

Egg, 40-43, 46, 49, 56-58, 64-65, 72-73, 76, 87, 105-107

Ejaculation, 57-58, 88-89, 97, 106

Embryo, 46

Endocrine system, 87-88

Epididymis, 57

Erection, 58-59, 89

Estrogen, 64, 72, 87

Exhibitionist, 143, 165

Fallopian tube, 40, 43, 64, 72, 107

Family planning, 105, 164-165

Fetish, 143

Fetus, 46

Foreskin, 58

Gay, 128-129, 165. *See also* Homosexual

Gender, 8-11, 30, 48-49, 90, 127, 131-134

Genes, 41-42, 68, 87-89, 131

Glans, 58, 67

Gonorrhea, 80-81

Herpes simplex II, 81

Heterosexual, 81, 98, 129, 133-134, 137, 144

Homosexual, 81, 127-139, 142, 144. *See also* Gay

Hormones, 27-28, 56, 59, 64, 72, 88-89, 101, 107, 117, 120, 130, 167

Hymen, 66, 77

Incest, 144, 151-154, 156

Infertility, 49, 56

Intercourse, 9, 15-23, 31, 58, 65-66, 68, 81-84, 97-98, 104-105, 108, 128, 143, 151

Intra-uterine devices (IUD), 106, 108

Jock itch, 60

Kleptomania, 143

Labia majora, 67

Labia minora, 67

Labor, 49-51, 65

Leucorrhea, 65

Lust, 91, 95-96, 99, 102, 135, 145-146

Mammary glands, 68

Masochists, 144

Masturbation, 94-101

Maturity, 86, 114-115, 123-125

Meatus, 67

Menarche, 73-74, 87

Menopause, 64, 73

Menstruation, 65, 72-78, 87

Miscarriage, 47

Morning after pill, 107

Mucus plug, 65

Necrophilia, 144

Nocturnal emissions, 89

Norplant, 107

Nymphomaniac, 143

Onanism, 94

Orgasm, 56-58, 60, 65, 89, 97, 104, 106, 128, 131

Ovaries, 40, 42, 64, 72-73, 87

Ovulation, 87, 106

Ovum, 46, 64

Pedophilia, 143-144

Penis, 55-60, 65, 67, 82, 88-89, 97, 104, 106, 128

Period, 56, 72-75, 87-88

Pill, 106-108, 165

Pituitary gland, 87

Placenta, 43, 50

Playboy philosophy, 33

Pornography, 98, 144-145

Premature births, 48

Premenstrual syndrome (PMS), 75

Progesterone, 64, 72, 87

Prostate, 57

Prostitute, 132, 134, 144

Protected sex, 82-83

Puberty, 56, 59, 64, 68, 73, 87-88, 90, 130

Pubic hair, 66-67, 87

Pyromania, 143

Quicken, 45

Rape, 145-147

Repression, 34

Rh-negative factor, 47

Sadist, 144

Sanitary napkins, 65, 77

Scrotum, 55, 57, 60-61, 88

Seduce, 144, 153

Seduction, 144

Semen, 57-58, 67

Seminal vesicles, 57, 89

Sexist, 30

Sexual deviation, 142-148

Sexual freedom, 32-33, 168

Sexuality, 8-12, 15-17, 20, 22-23, 25-26, 31, 33-37, 83-84, 90, 138-139, 148, 165, 167-168

Sexually transmitted diseases (STD), 80, 82, 144, 146, 164

Sperm, 40-42, 48-49, 55-58, 60, 64-65, 83, 89-90, 104-106, 108, 146

Spermatic cords, 55

Spermicides, 104

Sponges, 105

Stereotype, 29

Sterilization, 105

Syphilis, 80-81, 164

Tampons, 66, 76-78

Testes, 55, 57

Testicle, 55-57, 60, 88

Testosterone, 56, 64

Transsexual, 129

Transvestite, 130

Twins, 42, 165

Umbilical cord, 43-44, 50-51

Unisex, 26

Urethra, 57-58, 67

Uterus, 40, 43, 46, 50, 65, 72, 76, 106

Vagina, 40, 50, 58-59, 65-67, 77, 97, 104-106

Vaginal infection, 66

Vas deferens, 57

Venereal disease (VD), 80-81, 83, 105, 164

Voyeurs, 143

Vulva, 66

Water breaking, 50

Wet dreams, 59, 89-90

Withdrawal, 106

Womb, 40, 43, 45, 48-51, 63, 65, 68, 78, 106, 109

Zygote, 46